W0043246

Simulation Training for Obstetric Emergencies in Low-Resource Countries

Cécile Monod • Irene Hoesli
Martina Gisin • Samira Akra
Annkathrin Butenschoen
Stavroula Katsaouni • Lara Sirdey Fiechter
Katharina Redling

Simulation Training for Obstetric Emergencies in Low-Resource Countries

Practical Manual

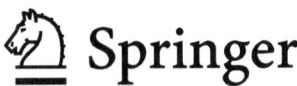 Springer

Cécile Monod, MD
Department of Obstetrics and
Feto-Maternal Medicine
University Hospital Basel
Basel, Switzerland

Martina Gisin, MSc
Department of Health Professions
Bern University of Applied Sciences
Bern, Switzerland

Department of Obstetrics and Antenatal Care
University Hospital Basel
Basel, Switzerland

Annkathrin Butenschoen, MD
Department of Obstetrics and
Feto-Maternal Medicine
University Hospital Basel
Basel, Switzerland

Lara Sirdey Fiechter, MD
Department of Obstetrics and
Feto-Maternal Medicine
University Hospital Basel
Basel, Switzerland

Irene Hoesli, Prof.em.
Basel University
Basel, Switzerland

Samira Akra, MD
Birth Center
Basel, Switzerland

Stavroula Katsaouni, MD
Department of Obstetrics and
Feto-Maternal Medicine
University Hospital Basel
Basel, Switzerland

Katharina Redling, MD
Department of Obstetrics and
Feto-Maternal Medicine
University Hospital Basel
Basel, Switzerland

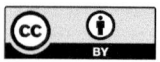

ISBN 978-3-031-81930-8   ISBN 978-3-031-81931-5   (eBook)
https://doi.org/10.1007/978-3-031-81931-5

Disclaimer: The dosage information and forms of application mentioned in this course manual have been checked with all due care, but no guarantee can be given for their correctness. No liability claims can be made against the publisher.
Copyright: all right to the content of this manual belong to the authors. Its content is intended for personal use only.

© The Editor(s) (if applicable) and The Author(s) 2025, corrected publication 2025. This book is an open access publication.

Open Access This book is licensed under the terms of the Creative Commons Attribution 4.0 International License (http://creativecommons.org/licenses/by/4.0/), which permits use, sharing, adaptation, distribution and reproduction in any medium or format, as long as you give appropriate credit to the original author(s) and the source, provide a link to the Creative Commons license and indicate if changes were made.
The images or other third party material in this book are included in the book's Creative Commons license, unless indicated otherwise in a credit line to the material. If material is not included in the book's Creative Commons license and your intended use is not permitted by statutory regulation or exceeds the permitted use, you will need to obtain permission directly from the copyright holder.
The use of general descriptive names, registered names, trademarks, service marks, etc. in this publication does not imply, even in the absence of a specific statement, that such names are exempt from the relevant protective laws and regulations and therefore free for general use.
The publisher, the authors and the editors are safe to assume that the advice and information in this book are believed to be true and accurate at the date of publication. Neither the publisher nor the authors or the editors give a warranty, expressed or implied, with respect to the material contained herein or for any errors or omissions that may have been made. The publisher remains neutral with regard to jurisdictional claims in published maps and institutional affiliations.

This Springer imprint is published by the registered company Springer Nature Switzerland AG
The registered company address is: Gewerbestrasse 11, 6330 Cham, Switzerland

If disposing of this product, please recycle the paper.

Foreword

It is a great pleasure to present a short preface for this exceptional, most timely documentation and manual on 'Simulation Training for Obstetric Emergencies in Low- Resource Countries'. The manual is established on very practical long-term experience in clinical practice, public health consideration, simulation courses, and teaching/training efforts over the past decade in Somaliland, Tanzania, other LMICs, and also Northern settings.

The authors merit congratulations particularly as the manual not only is guiding health practitioners in low- and middle-income countries but also makes a more general contribution towards enhancing maternal and foetal health outcomes by reducing morbidity and mortality rates; thus, it also improves primary healthcare systems in Africa and similar contexts.

The book will become an essential tool in daily practice but will also find its way to key curricula through effective use in bedside teaching/training and discussions across different systems and cultures in all countries concerned. I strongly believe that the success of this manual is deeply rooted in the very practical, real-life basis of understanding, analysing, and building on realities of obstetrical emergencies in their real-life context. Moreover, the manual was established, well validated, and promoted through a joint, transcultural approach guided by partnership and the principle of 'mutual learning for change'. Consequently, the manual is adapted to immediate use and guidance as well as for in-depth analyses. The reader is pleasantly struck by its ease of use and the most useful guiding tables and figures. Thus, the manual becomes a wonderful companion to all involved in reproductive, maternal, and child health. I consider this manual as an essential contribution to our efforts in global public health as it documents the practical way forward in how societies can be changed, health can be improved, and poverty can be fought.

Finally, the manual highlights the importance of continual effort and commitment to maintaining and improving primary healthcare approaches—particularly for risk groups/populations—and how sustained commitment leads to achieving durable results. I wish you a stimulating and enjoyable reading as well as a continued use and application for the benefit of those most in need.

Swiss Tropical & Public Health   Marcel Tanner, Prof.em.
Institute (Swiss TPH)
University Basel
Basel, Switzerland

Acknowledgements

We thank all those who have inspired and supported the development of this manual for simulation of obstetrical emergencies in low-income countries.

We are deeply grateful to the midwives and doctors from Kitete Referral Hospital, Tabora, Tanzania, and Edna Adan Hospital, Hargeisa, Somaliland, and all the participants from the simulation courses. Your input and your experiences have inspired this initiative and helped us in designing this manual.

Our sincere thanks also go to the University Hospital Basel, Switzerland, who provided the financial support necessary for this project. Your contributions ensure that this manual reaches those who need it most, empowering healthcare workers to act with confidence and precision during obstetrical emergencies.

The original version of the book has been revised. A correction to this book can be found at https://doi.org/10.1007/978-3-031-81931-5_12

Contents

List of Figures

List of Tables

Chapter 1
Introduction

This course manual provides the theoretical basis of the simulation course in obstetric emergencies made available in sub-Saharan countries by the dedicated obstetric team for mother-child projects of the University Hospital Basel in Africa. It provides midwives and doctors with addition information regarding the practical parts of the course and the different simulation scenarios. This document is the first version of this manual and is a 'work in progress' that will be enriched and updated in further versions. We are thankful for any comments or specific requests regarding the content, which can be addressed to the corresponding author.

Open Access This chapter is licensed under the terms of the Creative Commons Attribution 4.0 International License (http://creativecommons.org/licenses/by/4.0/), which permits use, sharing, adaptation, distribution and reproduction in any medium or format, as long as you give appropriate credit to the original author(s) and the source, provide a link to the Creative Commons license and indicate if changes were made.

The images or other third party material in this chapter are included in the chapter's Creative Commons license, unless indicated otherwise in a credit line to the material. If material is not included in the chapter's Creative Commons license and your intended use is not permitted by statutory regulation or exceeds the permitted use, you will need to obtain permission directly from the copyright holder.

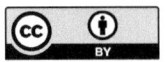

© The Author(s) 2025
C. Monod et al., *Simulation Training for Obstetric Emergencies in Low-Resource Countries*, https://doi.org/10.1007/978-3-031-81931-5_1

Chapter 2
Non-technical Skills

2.1 Introduction

Key Learning Points
- Non-technical skills (NTS) are cognitive and social skills that support technical skills in the execution of complex tasks which are necessary within a team for safe and effective management of emergency situations.
  They are skills for communication, teamwork and leadership, correctly assessing the situation and making appropriate decisions.
- Poor NTS within a team, such as poor teamwork and communication, are mostly responsible for avoidable adverse events and maternal deaths in maternity care.
- Frequent problems include the following:
  - Calling for help too late.
  - Failing to recognize the severity of the woman's condition.
  - Failing to communicate the severity of the woman's condition to all members of the team.

Effective management of obstetric emergencies requires the coordinated action of a team of caregivers composed of midwives, nurses and medical officers and doctors. Obstetric emergencies are often unforeseeable, and every team taking care of pregnant women should be prepared to respond rapidly and adequately. Obstetric emergencies are very stressful events for the women as well as for the team. Although an excellent command of technical skills is a prerequisite to managing these situations, NTS are also essential. NTS are social and cognitive skills that are necessary for safe and effective performance [1]. They include teamwork, communication, situation awareness, and task management within the team. High-risk industries, particularly aviation, have recognized the importance of training their crews to manage NTS since the late 1970s. Investigations of aircraft accidents showed that 70% of them involved NTS [2]. Implementing specific training for NTS led to a decrease in adverse events in aviation [3]. NTS play an essential role in avoidable adverse events in maternity care. National reports in the United Kingdom recognized

© The Author(s) 2025
C. Monod et al., *Simulation Training for Obstetric Emergencies in Low-Resource Countries*, https://doi.org/10.1007/978-3-031-81931-5_2

problems in communication and teamwork as a cause of preventable maternal deaths and neonatal asphyxia [4]. In particular, problematic communication and teamwork led junior team members to seek senior support too late, and teams failed to recognize and communicate the severity of the woman's condition to all members of the obstetric team. In this chapter, you will learn about useful tools for effectively communicating within your team in emergencies and beyond.

2.2 Situation Awareness: 'Helicopter View'

Situation awareness means being aware of what is happening around you in terms of where you are, where you are supposed to be, and whether anyone or anything around you is a threat to your health and safety. In case of an obstetric emergency, this means being aware of the severity of the woman's condition and how this condition is evolving. This is an essential step in planning to manage the situation properly and anticipating potential errors and threats. Situation awareness is also called helicopter view, because it reflects a broad rather than a narrowly focussed awareness. In a seminar on visual awareness, Simons et al. could analyse the knowledge that an unexpected event might occur does not increase the likelihood that people will notice other unexpected events (Fig. 2.1) [5].

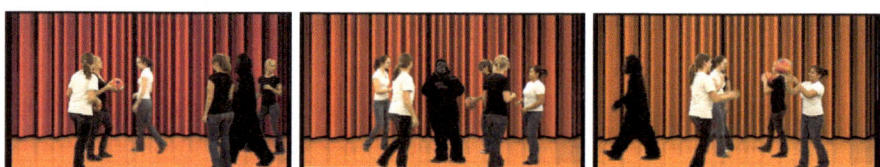

Fig. 2.1 Monkey business illusion [5]. (With permissions from Daniel Simons)

2.3   Communication Techniques That Help Maintain Situation Awareness

We are all human: We all make mistakes. Some communication techniques can help us avoid them by maintaining situation awareness:

• Call for help
• Use closed-loop communication
• Speak up
• Take the lead

Using *closed-loop communication*, the person receiving instructions or information repeats it back to make sure the message is understood correctly, and the sender confirms to 'close the loop'. It does not require more time, and in fact, it is likely to save time. But ultimately, it is an important tool that protects patients from communication errors that can lead to serious consequences.

Speaking up means that each member of the team should voice their concerns aloud.

Taking the lead refers to one team member adopting the role of team leader and keeping an overview of the situation. Most of the time, it will be the more experienced team member but if this person is busy, another one should take the lead.

Five signs that you are losing situational awareness:

• You feel confused.
• You feel increasingly stressed.
• You are experiencing conflict within the team.
• You discover key information has been missed.
• Something just does not feel right.

2.4   CRM

CRM stays for Crew Resource Management and has been adapted from aviation. It is a practical method to overcome communication failures, avoid human errors, or mitigate the consequences of error in emergency situations [6]. As we often hurry up in an emergency situation, we might oversee important facts. The 10 for 10 concept means that 10 s more in data gathering, diagnosing, and team planning, you save time and improve safety for the next 10 min or more for the patient. Rall et al. summarized the most important key points [7].

1. Know the environment
2. Anticipate and plan
3. Call for help early
4. Exercise leadership and followership with assertiveness
5. Distribute the workload (10-for 10 concept)

6. Mobilize all available resources
7. Communicate effectively—speak up
8. Use all available information
9. Prevent and manage fixation errors
10. Cross double check (never assume anything)
11. Use cognitive aids (algorithm)
12. Re-evaluate repeatedly (10-for 10-concept)
13. Use good teamwork, coordinate with, and support others
14. Allocate attention wisely
15. Set priorities dynamically

2.5   SBAR

SBAR is the acronym for situation/background/assessment/recommendation. This is a tool for communicating effectively and rapidly between providers and clearly states what the concern is and allows the individual communicating to make a strong recommendation for action [8] (Fig. 2.2).

SBAR report to clinician about a clinical obstetric situation

S	**Situation**
	I am calling about (woman's name): _____ Ward: _____ Hosp No: _____
	The problem I am calling about is: _____
	I have just made an assessment:
	The vital signs are: Blood pressure ____/____ Pulse ____ Respirations_____ SPO$_2$ _____% Temperature_____^{0}C

I am concerned about:	
Blood pressure because it is:	**Maternal serum lactate** because it is:_____mmol/l
systolic over 160	
diastolic over 100	**Urine output** because it is:
systolic less than 90	less than 100mls over the last 4 hours
Pulse because it is:	significantly proteinuric (+++)
over 120	**Haemorrhage:**
less than 40	Antepartum
Respirations because they are:	Postpartum
less than 10	**Fetal wellbeing:**
over 30	Pathological CTG
The woman is having oxygen at	**FBS Result:** pH _____
_____ l/min	Time sample taken: _____ hrs
Maternal temperature because it is: ___^{0}C	
	Obstetric Early Warning Chart Score: ▢ ▢

B	**Background** (tick relevant sections)

The woman is:
Primparous   Multiparous   Grand multparous
Gestation: _____ wks   Singleton   Multiple
Previous Caesarean section or uterine surgery
Fetal wellbeing
Abdominal palpation:
Fundal height:_____cms   Presentation:_____ Fifths palpable: _____ FH rate:_____bpm
CTG: Normal   Suspicious   Pathological
Antenatal
A/N problem (details): _____
Labour
Spontaneous onset   Induced
IUGR   Pre eclampsia   Reduced Fetal movements   Diabetes   APH
Syntocinon
Most recent vaginal examination: Time _____hrs
Cervical dilatation: _____cms   Station of presenting part: _____   Position: _____
Membranes intact   Meconium stained liquor   Fresh red loss PV
Third stage complete   Retained placenta
Postnatal
Delivery date: _____ Delivery time:_____hrs
Type of delivery:_____   Perineal trauma:_____
Blood loss: _____mls   Syntocinon infusion
Fundus: High   Atonic   Uterus tender   Abdominal/perineal wound oozing

Treatment given / in progress:_____

A	**Assessment**
	I think the problem is: _____
	I am not sure what the problem is but the woman is deteriorating and we need to do something

R	**Recommendation**
	Request:
	Please come to see the woman immediately
	I think delivering needs to be expedited
	I think the woman needs to be transferred to delivery suite
	I would like advice please
	Reported to: _____ **Response:** _____

Person completing form (name):_____Date:_____ Time: _____

Fig. 2.2 SBAR (PROMPT) [9]. (Reproduced with permission of the Licensor through PLSclear)

2.6 Conclusion

Effective teamwork and communication within the team are essential to the successful management of obstetric emergencies.

References

1. Gordon M, Baker P, Catchpole K, Darbyshire D, Schocken D. Devising a consensus definition and framework for non-technical skills in healthcare to support educational design: a modified Delphi study. Med Teach. 2015;37(6):572–7.
2. Helmreich RL. On error management: lessons from aviation. BMJ. 2000;320(7237):781–5.
3. Haerkens MH, Kox M, Lemson J, Houterman S, van der Hoeven JG, Pickkers P. Crew resource management in the intensive care unit: a prospective 3-year cohort study. Acta Anaesthesiol Scand. 2015;59(10):1319–29.
4. Knight M, Kenyon S, Brocklehurst P, Neilson J, Shakespeare J, Kurinczuk JJ, editors. On behalf of MBRRACEUK. Saving lives, improving mothers' care—lessons learned to inform future maternity care from the UK and Ireland confidential enquiries into maternal deaths and morbidity 2009–12. Oxford: National Perinatal Epidemiology Unit, University of Oxford; 2014.
5. Simons DJ. Monkeying around with the gorillas in our midst: familiarity with an inattentional-blindness task does not improve the detection of unexpected events. Iperception. 2010;1(1):3–6.
6. Nielsen P, Mann S. Team function in obstetrics to reduce errors and improve outcomes. Obstet Gynecol Clin N Am. 2008;35(1):81–95, ix.
7. Rall MGD. Human performance and patient safety. In: Miller's anesthesia. Philadelphia: Elsevier, Churchill Livingstone; 2009. p. 93–150.
8. Haig KM, Sutton S, Whittington J. SBAR: a shared mental model for improving communication between clinicians. Jt Comm J Qual Patient Saf. 2006;32(3):167–75.
9. The PROMPT Editorial Team. PROMPT course manual, practical obstetric multi-professional training. 3rd ed. Cambridge University Press; 2017.

Open Access This chapter is licensed under the terms of the Creative Commons Attribution 4.0 International License (http://creativecommons.org/licenses/by/4.0/), which permits use, sharing, adaptation, distribution and reproduction in any medium or format, as long as you give appropriate credit to the original author(s) and the source, provide a link to the Creative Commons license and indicate if changes were made.

The images or other third party material in this chapter are included in the chapter's Creative Commons license, unless indicated otherwise in a credit line to the material. If material is not included in the chapter's Creative Commons license and your intended use is not permitted by statutory regulation or exceeds the permitted use, you will need to obtain permission directly from the copyright holder.

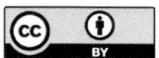

Chapter 3
Maternal Cardiac Arrest

3.1 Introduction: Background and Evidence

Key Learning Points
- Recognizing maternal cardiac arrest.
- Assessment and management
  - Evaluating ABC: **A**irway–**B**reathing–**C**irculation.
  - Performing basic life support: cardiac compression and ventilation (breathing).
  - Performing uterine displacement to the left (manual or 15–30° tilt; avoid/release aortocaval compression).
- Common issues include
  - Not calling for help.
  - Not starting basic life support (cardiac compression and ventilation)
  - Not performing uterine displacement to the left.
  - Not giving oxygen to the woman.

Definition
What do we mean by 'maternal cardiac arrest'? Maternal cardiac arrest is sometimes also described as 'maternal collapse'. In this situation, the woman's heartbeat suddenly stops, and the woman will become unconscious, not responding to voice or pain. She will not be breathing anymore—a situation called respiratory arrest—when she suffers cardiac arrest.

The occurrence of maternal cardiac arrest is rare, and survival is low. Its management is complicated in pregnant women by the physiological changes in pregnancy. A maternal cardiac arrest may be reversible in certain circumstances. To have a chance of survival, resuscitation manoeuvres must be started within a few minutes of the occurrence of cardiac arrest and a reversible cause identified and treated as soon as possible. Cardiac arrest leads to hypoxia, irreversible brain damage, and death in a short time—within minutes. Therefore, starting resuscitation manoeuvres

© The Author(s) 2025
C. Monod et al., *Simulation Training for Obstetric Emergencies in Low-Resource Countries*, https://doi.org/10.1007/978-3-031-81931-5_3

immediately is crucial—**first chest compression**—although other manoeuvres are also essential.

Causes of Maternal Cardiac Arrest Include [1]
- Haemorrhage
- Pre-eclampsia/eclampsia
- Pulmonary embolism
- Amniotic fluid embolism
- Sepsis
- Magnesium toxicity
- Total spinal anaesthesia
- Local anaesthetic toxicity

In addition, other causes of cardiac arrest in non-pregnant adults also apply to pregnant and postpartum women, such as cardiac disease, anaphylaxis (severe allergic reaction), and trauma, among others.

Specificity of Maternal Cardiopulmonary Resuscitation [1]
Physiological changes that hinder effective cardiopulmonary resuscitation in pregnant women are as follows:
- Compression of the aorta and vena cava (aortocaval compression) by the gravid uterus can occur in the supine position, diminishing the amount of blood pumped by each cardiac contraction (Fig. 3.1).
- Pulmonary residual capacity (pulmonary volume that is available for gas exchange) is reduced by 20% at the end of pregnancy. At the same time there is an increase in demand for oxygen of 20%.

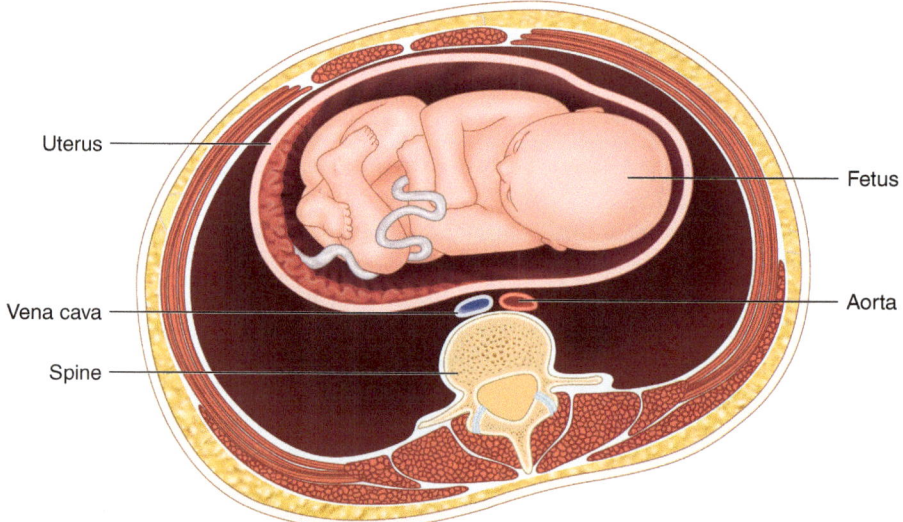

Fig. 3.1 Aorta and vena cava compression in supine position

- For this reason, pregnant women develop hypoxia more rapidly than non-pregnant women.
- The risk of pulmonary aspiration of gastric contents, which is complicated by difficult oxygenation as well as infectious complications, is also increased in pregnancy.

Although most general principles of adult cardiopulmonary resuscitation apply to pregnant women and those who just gave birth, some specificities must be considered in the management of maternal cardiac arrest because of the physiological changes.

3.1.1 General Principles

3.1.1.1 Manual Uterine Displacement to the Left

To allow for effective cardiopulmonary resuscitation, the woman should lie on a firm surface in the supine position. To relieve aortocaval compression by the gravid uterus, an assistant should perform **manual displacement of the uterus to the left**. Alternatively, the woman can be tilted 15–30° to the left side. However, if possible, it is preferable to choose manual uterine displacement to the left as rescucitation manoeuvres will be easier to perform effectively.

3.1.1.2 ABC General Principles

When encountering a pregnant woman (or any other person) who is non-responsive or unconscious, always use a systematic assessment: ABC.

Assess airway (A), before breathing (B), before circulation (C)
If the woman is not breathing, cardiac arrest should be assumed and cardiopulmonary resuscitation immediately started. Experienced clinicians may try to palpate a pulse. However, this can be very challenging and should not postpone first resuscitation measures. **Give 30 chest compressions** followed by two ventilations (breaths with face mask or mouth-to-mouth breath). This is called Basic Life Support or BLS.

3.1.1.3 Perimortem Caesarean Section

A perimortem birth is a birth that is expedited within **5 min** of maternal cardiac arrest. It releases aortocaval compression and allows for better lung ventilation and oxygenation of the woman. If the foetal station is below the spine, then operative vaginal birth may be an option. If the foetal station is higher, then perform a perimortem caesarean section. A scalpel is the minimal equipment that is needed to perform it. The objective of perimortem birth is primarily to improve the mother's chances of survival but it can also save the child.

3.1.2   Basic Life Support

Figure 3.2 presents the measures that should immediately be performed when a pregnant woman (or any other adult, omitting displacement of the uterus to the left) is found unconscious and has had a cardiac arrest.

3.1.2.1   How to Recognize Cardiac Arrest?

- A person is found unresponsive with absent or abnormal breathing.
- Slow, laboured breathing (agonal breathing) should be considered a cardiac arrest.
- ⟶ Start chest compressions as soon as possible.

Table 3.1 describes the step-by-step advanced management of the pregnant woman with cardiac arrest in a hospital setting.

Fig. 3.2 Cardiopulmonary resuscitation in the pregnant woman. (Copyright European Resuscitation Council, www.erc.edu, 2024_ NGL_028 [2])

BASIC LIFE SUPPORT

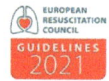

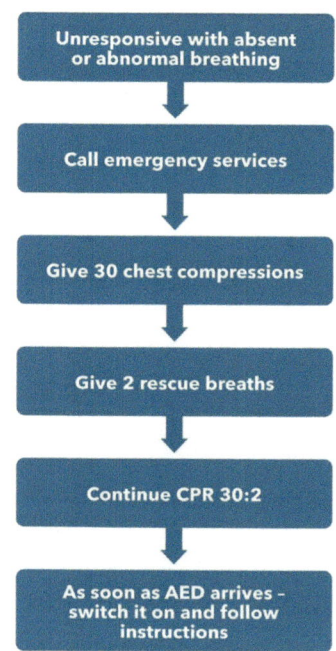

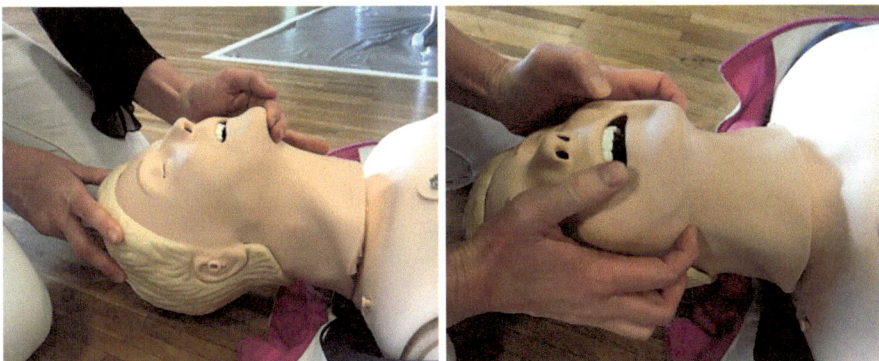

Fig. 3.3 Manoeuvres to open airways

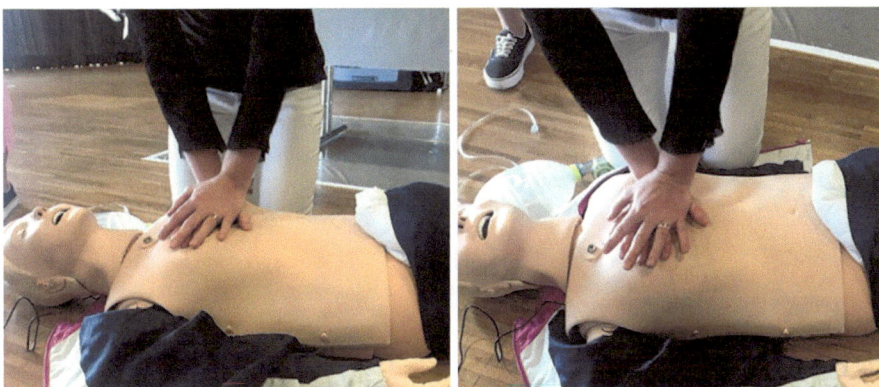

Fig. 3.4 Chest compression

Table 3.1 Step-by-step advanced management of the pregnant woman with cardiac arrest in a hospital setting (adapted from [3, 4])

Step	Details
Safety	Ensure safety of yourself, the woman, and helpers
Help	Call/shout for help (midwife, nurse, obstetrician, anaesthetist, paediatrician)
Response	Shake gently, ask loudly: 'Do you hear me? Are you all right'? A woman responding in a normal voice is assumed to have an open airway, normal breathing, and normal brain perfusion
A: Airway Open the airway	If not responding, lay the woman on her back on a firm surface. If on a bed: lay the bed flat and remove soft mattress **Manual displacement of uterus to the left by an assistant** Open the mouth, check for debris/foreign bodies Open airway: • Chin lift: Lift the chin with your fingertips or • Jaw thrust: Place fingers behind the angle of the jaw and displace the jaw anteriorly (Fig. 3.3) • If trauma is suspected, stabilization of cervical spine by an assistant

(continued)

Table 3.1 (continued)

Step	Details
B: Breathing Look, listen, feel for breathing	Assess breathing for no more than 10 s: • Look/palpate for chest movements • Listen for abnormal sounds indicating pharyngeal or laryngeal obstruction • Feel air flow through mouth and nose on expiration ➡ If absent breathing, woman is assumed to have cardiac arrest (see C)
C: Circulation	Assess carotid pulse (only for experienced team, challenging) **Manual displacement of uterus to the left** (should be done as soon as possible, already when assessing airway) Begin **cardiopulmonary resuscitation (CPR)** without delay (Fig. 3.4): • Place the heel of the hand in the centre of the thorax (lower half of breastbone) • Place the heel of the other hand on top of the first hand • Keep your arms straight • Position yourself vertically above the woman's chest • Compress the chest to a depth of 5–6 cm • Release the pressure • Repeat at a rate of 100–120 compressions/min • Give 2 breaths (with a ventilation mask or mouth-to-mouth breath). Do not interrupt chest compressions for >10 s for the 2 breaths • If available, give breaths by ventilation mask with 100% oxygen (Fig. 3.5) • Continue at a rate of 30 chest compression for 2 breaths • Take turns for chest compressions every 2 min (exhausting task) If in hospital: Ensure intravenous access with at least one large bore cannula
Expedite birth within 5 min of unsuccessful CPR	Prepare for perimortem birth: caesarean section (ask for a scalpel) or operative vaginal birth depending on foetal station CPR to be continued throughout procedure Once resuscitation has been successful, move to the operating theatre to close the uterus and abdomen if caesarean section has been done. Be prepared to manage massive postpartum haemorrhage
Think 4Hs and 4Ts (Table 3.2)	Correct reversible causes of maternal cardiac arrest
Cessation of resuscitation	In case of unsuccessful resuscitation, the decision to abandon it should be taken by the most experienced clinician available in consultation with the rest of the team
After events	Explain the situation and what has been done in all case with the woman, if she survived, and with relatives and the team afterwards

Table 3.2   Possible reversible causes of maternal cardiac arrest [1]

4Hs	4Ts
Hypoxia	Thromboembolic disease • Pulmonary embolism • Amniotic fluid embolism
Hypovolaemia	Tension pneumothorax
Hypothermia	Therapeutic or toxic • Inadvertent intravenous administration of local anaesthetics • Opioid overdose
Hyperkalaemia and other metabolic disorders like hypoglycaemia	Cardiac Tamponade

Fig. 3.5 Ventilation mask

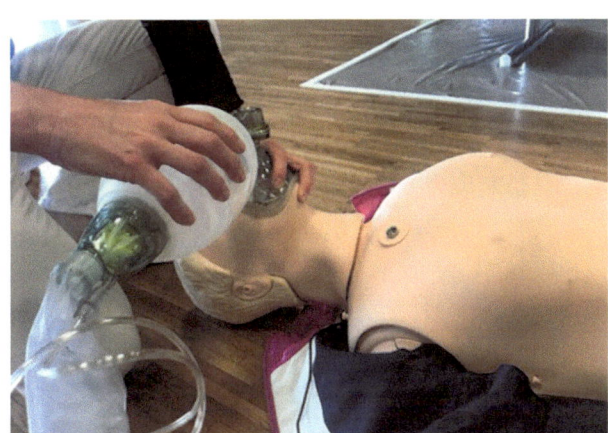

Do Not Forget

Perform manual uterine displacement to the left to relieve aortocaval compression!
Continue cardiopulmonary resuscitation throughout perimortem caesarean section or operative vaginal birth!
Expedite the birth within 5 min of maternal cardiac arrest!

3.2   Algorithm

Figure 3.6 depicts the algorithm for addressing maternal cardiac arrest.

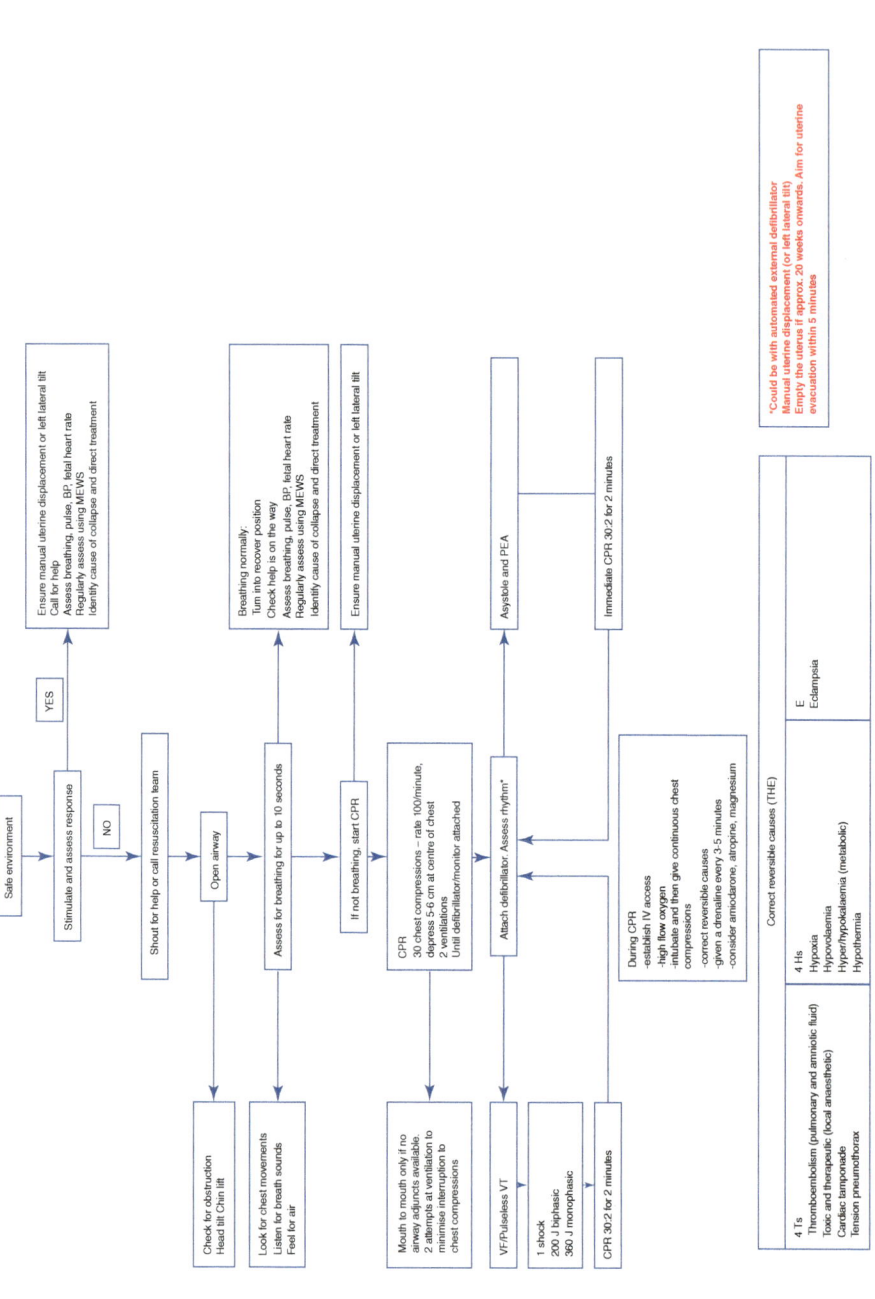

Fig. 3.6 Maternal resuscitation [1]. (Reproduced from: Chu J, Johnston TA, Geoghegan J, on behalf of the Royal College of Obstetricians and Gynaecologists. Maternal Collapse in Pregnancy and the Puerperium. BJOG 2020;127:e14–e52, with the permission of the College)

3.3 Conclusion

Maternal cardiac arrest is a rare event. Unless managed within a very short time, it will inevitably lead to death. Recognizing cardiac arrest is a crucial skill and can be achieved with a systematic evaluation—ABC—within seconds. Resuscitation specificities exist in pregnant women because of pregnancy-related physiological changes and should be managed appropriately displacing the uterus to the left and proceeding to perimortem birth to improve maternal survival chances within 5 min of cardiac arrest.

References

1. Chu J, Johnston TA, Geoghegan J. Maternal collapse in pregnancy and the puerperium: greentop guideline no. 56. BJOG. 2020;127(5):e14–52.
2. Olasveengen TM, Semeraro F, Ristagno G, Castren M, Handley A, Kuzovlev A, et al. European Resuscitation Council Guidelines 2021: basic life support. Resuscitation. 2021;161:98–114.
3. Gandhi A, Gandhi A. Cardiopulmonary resuscitation in the pregnant woman. Global Women's Medicine; 2021. p. 13.
4. Burns R, Dent K. Managing medical and obstetric emergencies and trauma. The MOET course manual. 4th ed. Cambridge University Press; 2022.

Open Access This chapter is licensed under the terms of the Creative Commons Attribution 4.0 International License (http://creativecommons.org/licenses/by/4.0/), which permits use, sharing, adaptation, distribution and reproduction in any medium or format, as long as you give appropriate credit to the original author(s) and the source, provide a link to the Creative Commons license and indicate if changes were made.

The images or other third party material in this chapter are included in the chapter's Creative Commons license, unless indicated otherwise in a credit line to the material. If material is not included in the chapter's Creative Commons license and your intended use is not permitted by statutory regulation or exceeds the permitted use, you will need to obtain permission directly from the copyright holder.

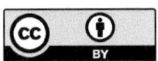

Chapter 4
Postpartum Haemorrhage

4.1 Introduction: Background and Evidence

Key Learning Points
- Understand risk factors, causes, and treatment of major obstetric haemorrhage.
- Perform early fluid resuscitation and do not delay blood transfusion based on a single haemoglobin value.
- Call for help, especially senior help, early.
- Understand the importance of 'accurately' measuring blood loss.
- Give tranexamic acid early as well as uterotonics.
- Consider hysterectomy if medical and surgical interventions are ineffective.

Definition

Postpartum haemorrhage (PPH; see Tables 4.1, 4.2 and 4.3) is still a leading direct cause of maternal death in both low- and high-income countries. PPH can be prevented by an active third stage of labour that means a prophylactic application of uterotonic (Oxytocin 10 IU IM or 5 IU IV) after cord clamping. Alternatively, heat stable Carbetocin (100 µg IM) can be used [2]. Active management of third stage of labour reduces mean maternal blood loss at birth and probably reduces the rate of primary blood loss greater than 500 mL and the use of therapeutic uterotonics [2, 3].

Timely and appropriate management of PPH saves maternal lives. Prompt recognition of the haemorrhage as well as efficient teamwork and communication is essential to manage the emergency.

Causes

The four Ts of PPH—tone, trauma, tissue, and thrombin—describe the most common causes (Table 4.4). Do not forget that more than one cause may be the origin of PPH.

Supplementary Information The online version contains supplementary material available at https://doi.org/10.1007/978-3-031-81931-5_4.

© The Author(s) 2025, corrected publication 2025
C. Monod et al., *Simulation Training for Obstetric Emergencies in Low-Resource Countries*, https://doi.org/10.1007/978-3-031-81931-5_4

Table 4.1 Definition of PPH [1]

Postpartum haemorrhage
• Blood loss of 500 mL or more from the genital tract within 24 h of the birth of a baby (vaginal birth) • Blood loss of >1000 mL from the genital tract within 24 h after caesarean section • Blood loss accompanied by signs or symptoms of hypovolaemia within 24 h after birth

Table 4.2 Definition of PPH: primary versus secondary [1]

Definition of postpartum haemorrhage: primary versus secondary	
Level	Description
Primary	Loss of **500 mL or more** of blood from the genital tract within **24 h** of the birth of a baby
Secondary	Abnormal or excessive bleeding from the birth canal between 24 h and 12 weeks postnatally

Table 4.3 Definition of PPH: severity [1]

Severity of postpartum haemorrhage	
Level	Blood loss (mL)
Minor	500–1000
Major	>1000
Moderate	>1000–2000
Severe	>2000

Note. In women with lower body mass (body weight <60 kg), lower blood loss may already be clinically significant!

Table 4.4 Causes of PPH: the four Ts and concrete examples (*source*: Queensland Clinical Guidelines, Queensland Health © state of Queensland (Queensland Health) 2021 [4])

Four Ts (frequency)	Example
Tone (70%)	Atonic uterus
Trauma (20%)	Perineal, vaginal, cervical lacerations Extension tears of uterotomy at caesarean section Uterine rupture or inversion Non-genital-tract trauma (e.g. subcapsular liver rupture in HELLP, retroperitoneal haematoma)
Tissue (10%)	Retained placenta or remnants of placenta, membranes, or clots (always examine placenta after birth to control if it has been removed completely)
Thrombin (<1%)	Coagulation anomalies (e.g. in pre-eclampsia/eclampsia or HELLP, amniotic fluid embolism, maternal coagulopathy)

Note. HELLP **h**aemolysis, **e**levated **l**iver enzymes, **l**ow **p**latelets

Risk Factors

Recognizing risk factors for PPH beforehand enables risk stratification and better care. A pregnant woman presenting a high risk of PPH, for example, one who has a previous history of retained placenta and PPH, should be referred to give birth in a health care facility equipped to manage this complication. Although birth attendants

Table 4.5 Risk factors for PPH [5] (reproduced with permission of the Licensor through PLSclear)

Pre-labour

- Previous retained placenta or PPH (recurrence rate of about 8–10%)
- Previous caesarean section (associated with uterine rupture, placenta praevia, percreta and accreta)
- Placenta praevia, accreta or percreta
- Antepartum haemorrhage—especially from placental abruption
- Overdistension of uterus (e.g. multiple pregnancy, polyhydramnios, macrosomia)
- Pre-eclampsia
- Maternal weight below 60 kg (less able to tolerate blood loss due to smaller circulating volume)
- Body mass index above 35 kg/m^2
- Increased maternal age (in addition, older women are less tolerant of the effects of a massive bleeding)
- Existing uterine abnormalities (e.g. fibroids)
- Maternal haemoglobin below 90 g/L at start of labour (less able to tolerate haemorrhage and increased risk of uterine atony because of depleted uterine myoglobin levels necessary for muscle action)

Intrapartum

- Induction of labour
- Prolonged first, second or third stage of labour
- Use of oxytocin or misoprostol in labour (stimulating or augmenting uterine contractions should be performed in accordance with current guidance and should avoid uterine hyperstimulation)
- Retained placenta
- Precipitate labour
- Operative vaginal birth
- Caesarean section, particularly in the second stage of labour
- Placental abruption
- Pyrexia in labour

Remember: Anaemia is a risk factor for rapid haemodynamic decompensation if postpartum haemorrhage (PPH) occurs!

should always be prepared to manage PPH at every birth, being aware of the risk factors helps them refine the plan and not delay necessary interventions. Some risk factors appear during the birth. Significant risk factors for PPH are listed in Table 4.5.

4.2 Management

Figure 4.1 depicts a training exercise on managing PPH.

> Because of **frequent underestimation of blood loss**, PPH may first be recognized by symptoms of **haemodynamic decompensation**!

Fig. 4.1 Training exercise
on managing PPH

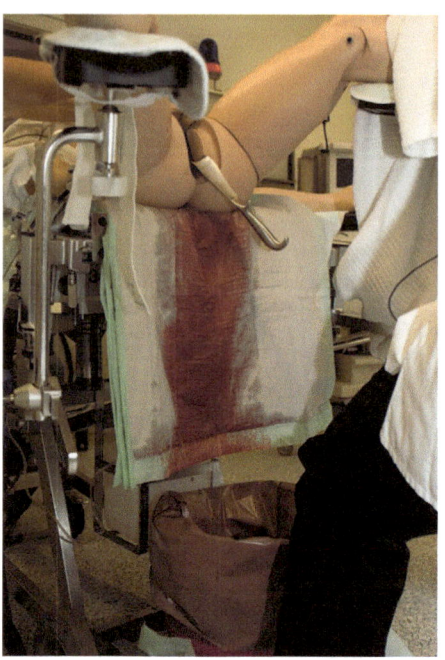

> **Delayed recognition of PPH** accounts for **maternal morbidity and mortality** in many situations!

4.2.1   Blood Loss Estimation

Maternal blood loss is often underestimated after birth, particularly in case of higher blood loss. In many cases, delayed recognition of PPH is responsible for maternal morbidity and mortality. Light but persistent bleeding may go unnoticed until the woman develops haemodynamic collapse, and its recognition may represent a particular challenge.

Any bleeding before birth and any amount of blood in towels, sanitary pads, or spilling onto the floor should be considered when estimating blood loss (Fig. 4.2). Remember that bleeding can be concealed within the uterus, broad ligament, or abdominal cavity, and the first presentation of PPH, in this case, may be a haemorrhagic shock. Tables 4.6, 4.7, and 4.8 mention key points to estimate blood loss correctly.

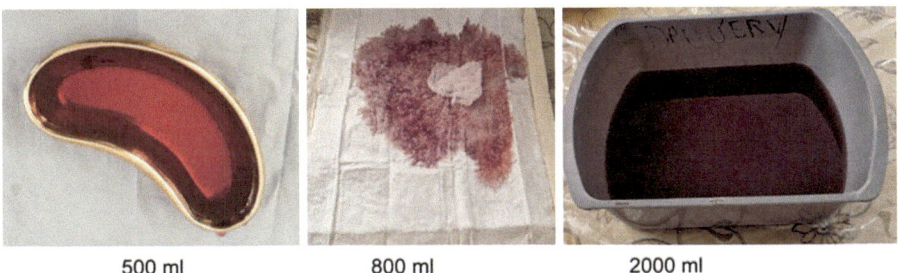

| 500 ml | 800 ml | 2000 ml |

Fig. 4.2 Blood loss estimation

Table 4.6 Blood loss estimation

- Weigh linen, swabs, drape, etc.
- Use visual pictograms
- Consider blood spilling onto the floor
- Consider antepartum blood loss
- Re-evaluate total blood loss at regular intervals
- If available, use a blood collection bag, Fig. 4.3

Table 4.7 Concealed haemorrhage

Do not forget concealed haemorrhage!
Bleeding can be concealed within the uterus, broad ligament, or abdominal cavity. First clinical signs in this case may be haemorrhagic shock.

4.2.2   Organization and Teamwork: Be Ready and Call for Help Early!

Successful management of PPH needs the action of a well-coordinated team. Calling for help too late is a frequent problem in managing PPH, leading to severe maternal morbidity and mortality. If simple actions cannot stop the bleeding, you should not hesitate to call for the help of an experienced midwife, obstetrician, and/or anaesthetist, if available. The laboratory should also be informed early in case a blood transfusion is needed. Effective communication within the team is essential, as effective management requires a series of parallel actions. It has proven very useful to have a so-called PPH box (Fig. 4.4) prepared in advance, which contains all necessary materials and drugs to treat the bleeding. It will save precious time when facing the emergency. It is also beneficial to have a chart within the PPH box with the dosage and administration route of available drugs.

Table 4.8 Signs of haemorrhagic shock and haemodynamic instability from [5] (reproduced with permission of the Licensor through PLSclear)

Blood loss	Clinical features	Level of shock
10% blood loss		
~500 mL if 50 kg	Mild tachycardia	Compensated
~800 mL if 80 kg	Normal blood pressure	
15% blood loss		
~750 mL if 50 kg	Tachycardia (>100 bpm)	Mild
~1200 mL if 80 kg	Hypotension (systolic 90–80 mmHg)	
	Tachypnoea (21–30 breaths/min)	
	Pallor, sweating	
	Weakness, faintness, thirst	
30% blood loss		
~1500 mL if 50 kg	Rapid, weak pulse (>120 bpm)	Moderate
~2400 mL if 80 kg	Moderate hypotension (systolic 80–60 mmHg)	
	Tachypnoea (>30 breaths/min)	
	Pallor, cold clammy skin	
	Poor urinary output (<30 mL/h)	
	Restlessness, anxiety, confusion	
40% blood loss		
~2000 mL if 50 kg	Rapid, weak pulse (>140 bpm) or bradycardia (<60 bpm)	Severe
~3200 mL if 80 kg	Severe hypotension (<70 mmHg)	
	Pallor, cold clammy skin, peripheral cyanosis	
	Air hunger	
	Anuria	
	Confusion or unconsciousness, collapse	

Note. Due to a higher blood volume in pregnancy, pulse rate and blood pressure are typically maintained until 30% of circulation volume is lost. Women may show no signs of haemodynamic decompensation until they have lost a large amount of blood but will then suddenly show signs of severe haemodynamic shock once compensatory mechanisms can no longer be maintained. Any raise in pulse rate or drop of blood pressure should prompt a clinical evaluation of blood loss. Do not rely on a single bedside measurement of haemoglobin or clotting factors [6]

4.2.3 Monitor the Woman

Check maternal blood pressure, pulse, temperature, and respiratory rate as well as urine output at regular intervals. By doing so, you will be aware of any ongoing changes in the state of the woman.

4.2.4 Search for the Cause of PPH: The Four Ts

Quickly perform a clinical assessment of the woman to identify the cause of the bleeding.

Fig. 4.3 Blood collection bag

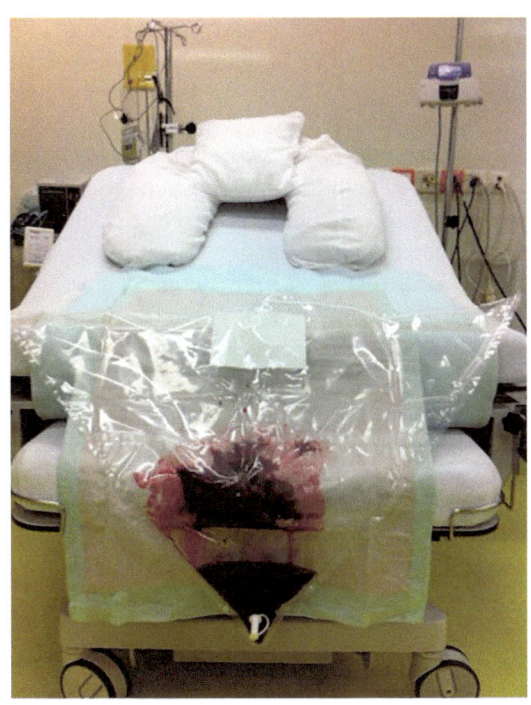

Fig. 4.4 PPH box containing all material and drugs needed to treat PPH

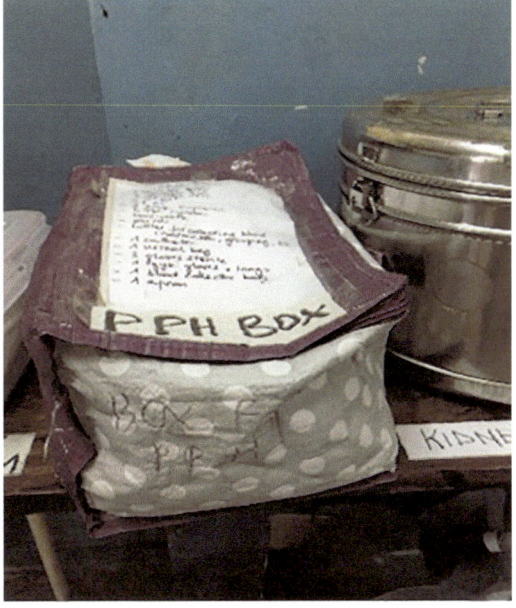

- *Palpate the uterus and assess the contraction.* Is it firm or soft? Does it contract with massage of the uterus, and does the bleeding stop? Can you expel clots? Note the position of the fundus above or below the umbilicus. Is the fundus higher than expected? Could it indicate concealed intrauterine bleeding or rupture?
- *Examine the birth canal.* Take care to expose the structures properly, with enough light and help from an assistant if needed. Give the woman adequate analgesics, which is essential for the woman's pain management and to allow you to perform an accurate examination. Examine the cervix and vagina for tears. Search for concealed vaginal haematoma by looking at and palpating the vaginal walls. Put clamps on and/or compress obvious vascular bleeding from the perineal lacerations until you can suture them.
- *Examine the placenta.* An assistant should perform this task whilst you are examining the woman. Is there any sign of incomplete placenta/retained products? If available, perform a quick abdominal ultrasound and look for intrauterine retained placenta cotyledons or intrauterine clot accumulation.

4.2.4.1   General Principles of Resuscitation: Acidosis–Coagulopathy–Hypovolaemia

Avoid Acidosis: Give Oxygen!

Lay the woman flat and give her oxygen with a face mask (10–15 L/min) to avoid acidosis.

Avoid Coagulopathy: Keep the Mother Warm!

Keeping the woman warm hinders the development of coagulopathy (blood not clotting properly anymore). Besides covering her with dry linens, warm the fluids you administer if possible.

4.2.4.2   Fluid and Blood Product Replacement: Correct Hypovolaemia and Coagulopathy!

To restore the circulating volume, you must administer crystalloid fluids such as normal saline quickly, up to 2000 mL. To quickly replace fluids, use two large cannulas of 18 (green) or 16 (grey) gauge. This allows a maximum flow of 90 mL/min (green) or 170 mL/min (grey). Establish intravenous (IV) access and use pressure bags. At some point, the woman will need a transfusion of packed red blood cells to restore oxygen carrying capacity and prevent her from developing a non-treatable haemorrhagic shock.

Coagulation must also be supported. The first-line drug is tranexamic acid, which should be administered early in the management of PPH if available. If the bleeding is strong and/or the woman is already in very severe haemorrhagic shock, do not wait for laboratory results such as haemoglobin or to crossmatch blood but transfuse O-negative blood.

4.2.5 Drugs for Treatment of PPH

Several drugs are available to treat PPH (Table 4.9).

4.2.6 Products to Support Coagulation

Several products are available to support coagulation (Table 4.10).

Table 4.9 Drugs of treatment of PPH

Drug	Administration	Mode of action/secondary effects
Oxytocin	10 IU IM or 5 IU IV (intravenous)	First choice, alternative to syntometrine
Syntometrine	Active third stage—give second dose IM (intramuscular) Physiological third stage—give first dose	Contraindicated with hypertension
Ergometrine	500 µg IM (if syntometrine has not been given)	Contraindicated with hypertension
Oxytocin infusion	20–40 IU in 1000 mL normal saline over 4 h	Will not initiate uterine contraction but may maintain it
Misoprostol	800 µg rectally	Secondary effects: shivering, pyrexia, diarrhoea Onset of action after 10 min, duration of action 4 h

Table 4.10 Products to support coagulation adapted from

Drug	Administration	Mode of action/secondary effects
Tranexamic acid	1 g IV May be repeated once in untreatable PPH not responding to treatment (max 2 g IV)	Prevents breakdown of fibrin and maintains blood clots. Reduction in maternal deaths from haemorrhage following vaginal or caesarean birth and reduction in women needing laparotomy to control bleeding. Should be administered early (optimally within 30 min) in PPH
Fresh frozen plasma (FFP) if available	For every 4 units FFP IV use 4 units of packed red cells	Liquid portion of whole blood. Contains coagulation factors but poor source of fibrinogen. Requires thawing (30 min)

4.2.7   Manual Removal of the Placenta

If the placenta is not delivered within 30 min after birth, be prepared for manual removal of the placenta. If the woman is not bleeding, you may wait for an additional 30 min (1 h after birth) for the placenta to deliver.

4.2.7.1   Before Starting the Procedure, You Should

- Give a second dose of oxytocin (5 IU, intramuscularly or intravenously) and perform a Credé manoeuvre (Fig. 4.5).
- Explain the procedure to the woman before performing the Credé manoeuvre.
- Ensure that the woman has an IV line in place. In case of heavy bleeding, put in a second IV line.
- Ensure the bladder is empty. If the woman cannot urinate, insert a urinary catheter with the usual aseptic technique.
- Give fluids.
- Give prophylactic antibiotics before starting the procedure according to your local protocols.

Fig. 4.5   Credé manoeuvre

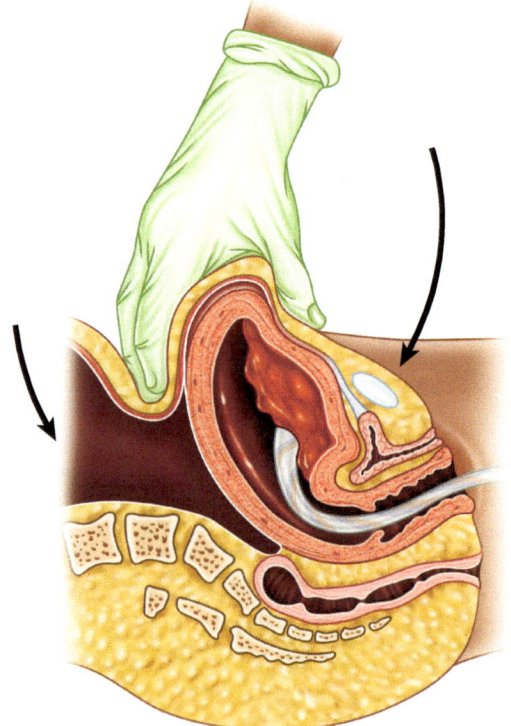

- Give an appropriate analgesic.
- Prepare an infusion with uterotonic, for example, 1 L normal saline with 20–40 IU oxytocin.
- <u>If</u> available, install a blood collection bag under the buttocks of the woman (Fig. 4.3).
- Disinfect the vulva and perineum with an antiseptic solution.

4.2.7.2   Technique for Manual Removal of the Placenta

- Wear sterile gloves.
- Support the uterine fundus with one hand on the abdomen to provide counter-pressure during manual removal and prevent uterine inversion.
- Follow the umbilical cord with the other hand through the cervix.
- Gently move your fingers to localize the edge of the placenta.
- Use gentle lateral and/or up and down movements of your fingers held tight together to find the cleavage plane between the placenta and the uterine wall.
- Sweep your fingers between the uterus wall and placenta and detach the placenta over its whole surface (Fig. 4.6).
- Hold the placenta in your hand and remove it slowly from the uterus.
- Palpate the uterine wall to ensure that placental tissue has been completely removed.

Fig. 4.6 Manual removal of the placenta

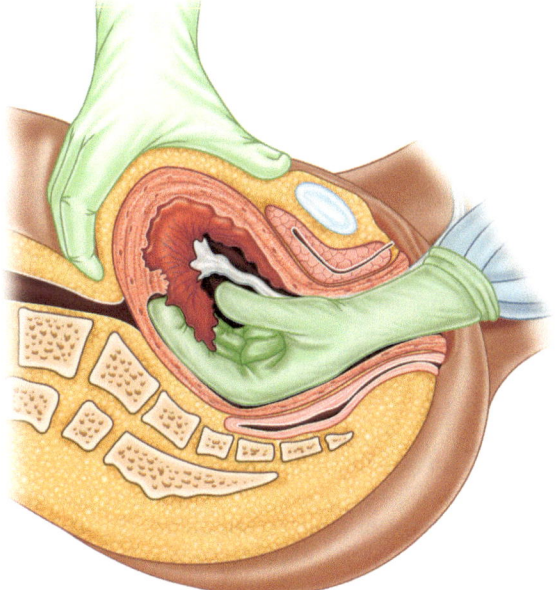

- If you suspect placental tissue remains, remove it by performing a gentle curettage with a blunted curette.

4.2.7.3 What to Do If the Placenta Does Not Detach with the Manual Removal Technique?

- If you cannot find the cleavage plane between the uterus and placenta, you should suspect placenta accreta, increta, or percreta. If the woman had previous caesarean deliveries, she has an increased risk of it. In these cases, discuss laparotomy.

4.2.7.4 What to Do If the Woman Is Bleeding Heavily During the Procedure?

- If available, send blood to the laboratory to check haemoglobin, thrombocytes, and coagulation.
- Be prepared to organize crossmatched packed red blood cells, or rhesus-negative blood if crossmatched is not readily available, to transfuse the woman if necessary.

4.2.8 Uterine and Aortic Compression

Whilst preparing to insert an intrauterine tamponade or transfer the woman to the operating theatre, you should ask another person to perform temporary manoeuvres to limit the amount of blood loss. One possibility is bimanual uterine compression and another is aortic compression, which are both very effective (Fig. 4.7).

4.2.9 Intrauterine Tamponade

To control refractory bleeding from the uterus, intrauterine tamponade techniques should be used. One consists of inserting an intrauterine balloon into the uterine cavity, as described below. Other options include packing the uterus with sterile gauzes attached together or inserting chitosan haemostatic gauze.

4.2.9.1 Intrauterine Balloon

A condom catheter inserted and inflated inside the uterus is an appropriate measure to control bleeding from uterine atony (Fig. 4.8). Give the woman sufficient analgesics and prophylactic antibiotics according to local protocol until balloon removal.

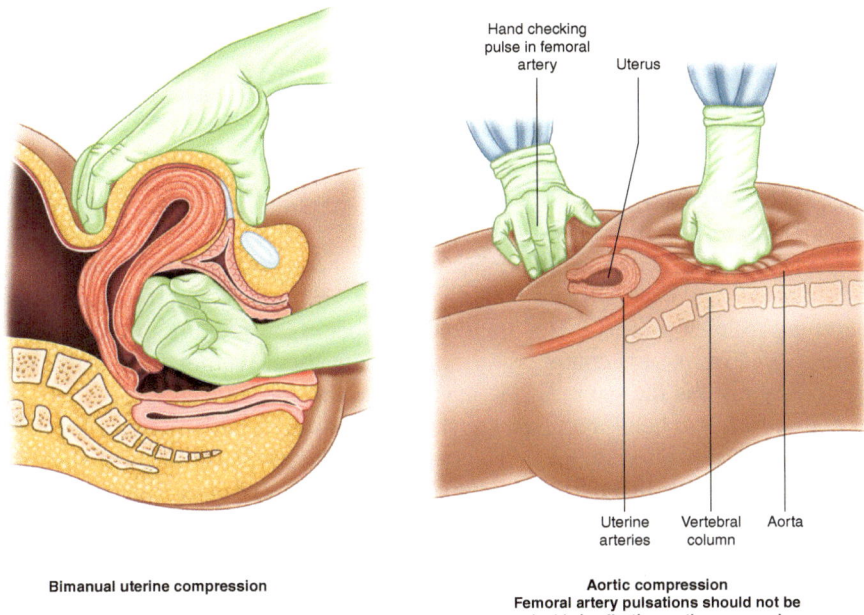

Bimanual uterine compression

Aortic compression
Femoral artery pulsations should not be palpable in effective aortic compression

Fig. 4.7 Temporary compression maoeuvres in PPH

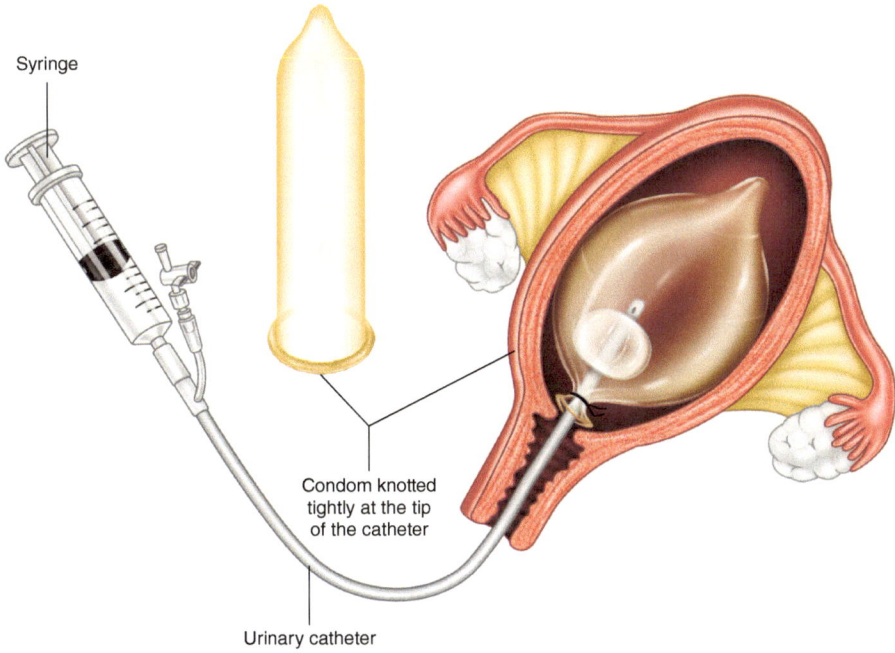

Fig. 4.8 Intrauterine balloon

Remove the balloon after maximal 24 h. The women should receive prophylactic antibiotics whilst the balloon is in place.

Detailed instructions on the procedure and materials are available on the platform of Global Health Media Project [7].

4.2.9.2   Uterus Packing

Sterile gauzes attached together are inserted into the uterine cavity to compress the placenta bed. Give the woman sufficient analgesics and prophylactic antibiotics according to local protocol. It is imperative to begin the packing in the fundus to achieve effective uterine compression. An assistant should stabilize the uterus from the abdomen. Pass the gauze to the hand inside the uterine cavity. You can use a dressing forceps to help you place the gauze but be careful not to pierce the uterus with your instruments (Fig. 4.9). The goal is to fill the uterine cavity with the gauze completely. Remove the gauze after maximal 24 h. The woman should receive prophylactic antibiotics whilst the packing is in place. Take care to count how many gauzes are inserted. Ensure that all gauzes have been removed from the uterus by counting them.

4.2.9.3   Celox® Gauze

Celox® gauze is a haemostatic gauze covered with chitosan, a product derived from crustaceans. It is a very effective alternative to an intrauterine balloon. Give the woman sufficient analgesics and prophylactic antibiotics according to local

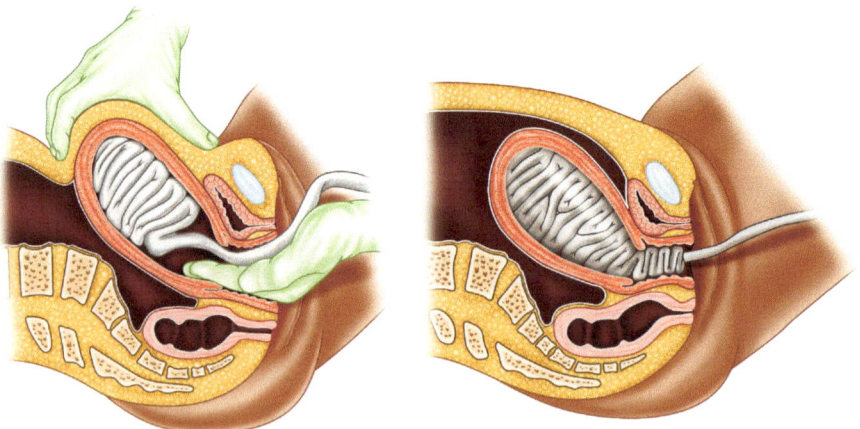

Sterile gauzes knotted together and inserted into the uterus cavity

Fig. 4.9 Uterine packing

protocol until gauze removal. Remove the Celox® gauze after maximal 24 h. The women should receive prophylactic antibiotics whilst the Celox® gauze is in place [8].

4.2.10 Operative Techniques

In case of persistent refractory bleeding, operative therapy is lifesaving. Several techniques have been described.

4.2.10.1 Haemostatic Brace Suturing

The objective of haemostatic brace suturing of the uterus is to achieve compression to stop the bleeding. Use a large, curved needle (catgut and polyglactin 910 sutures No. 1 or 2, 70 cm) with thick absorbable thread to go through the uterine wall. B-Lynch suture (Fig. 4.10) [9] should be performed with an open uterotomy, and Hayman sutures can be applied on a closed uterotomy (Fig. 4.11).

4.2.10.2 Uterine Artery Ligation

A stepwise uterine artery ligation may be performed to control the bleeding. For a more detailed technical description, please refer [10].

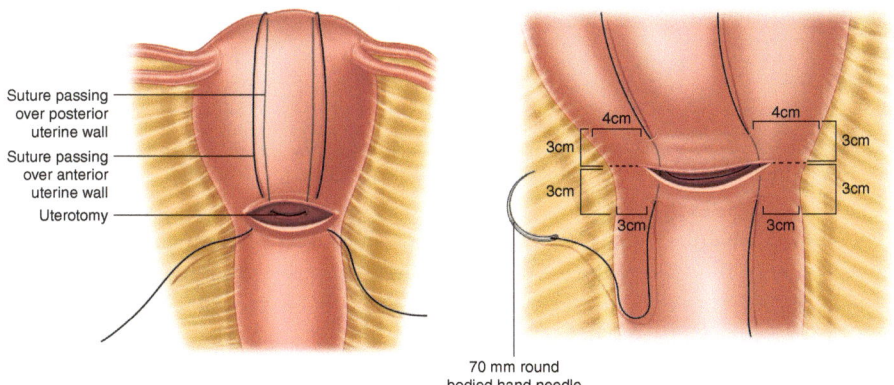

Fig. 4.10 B-Lynch haemostatic suture

Fig. 4.11 Hayman
haemostatic suture

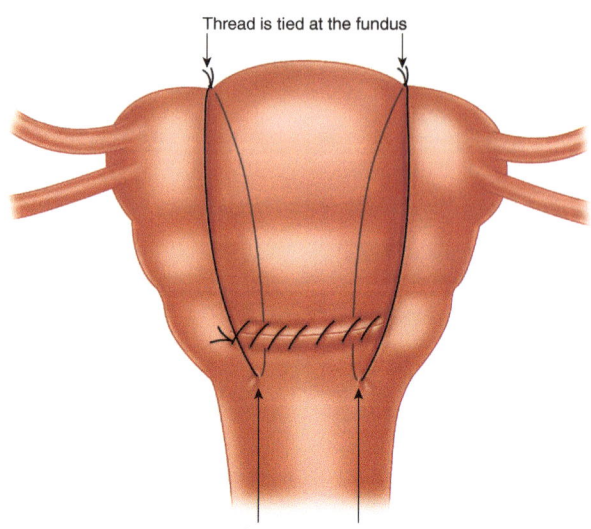

Thread is tied at the fundus

Transfixing the total uterine wall

4.2.10.3   Internal Iliac Artery Ligation

For a technical description of this technique, please refer [10].

4.2.10.4   Peripartum Hysterectomy

Peripartum hysterectomy should be seen as a last-resort manoeuvre in case of persistent and refractory bleeding. At the same time, peripartum hysterectomy may be a lifesaving procedure for the mother and should not be delayed until it is too late to save the woman. For a technical description, please refer to [11] or the following resource: [12].

4.3   Algorithm

The World Health Organization (WHO) has produced recommendations on the assessment of blood loss and a treatment bundle for postpartum haemorrhage [13].

The Jhpiego has an additional algorithm when PPH is refractory to all measures performed (Figs. 4.12 and 4.13).

The nonpneumatic antishock garment (NASG) reduces blood flow to the uterus by compressing and is as a temporary bridging measure until appropriate care is available (Fig. 4.14).

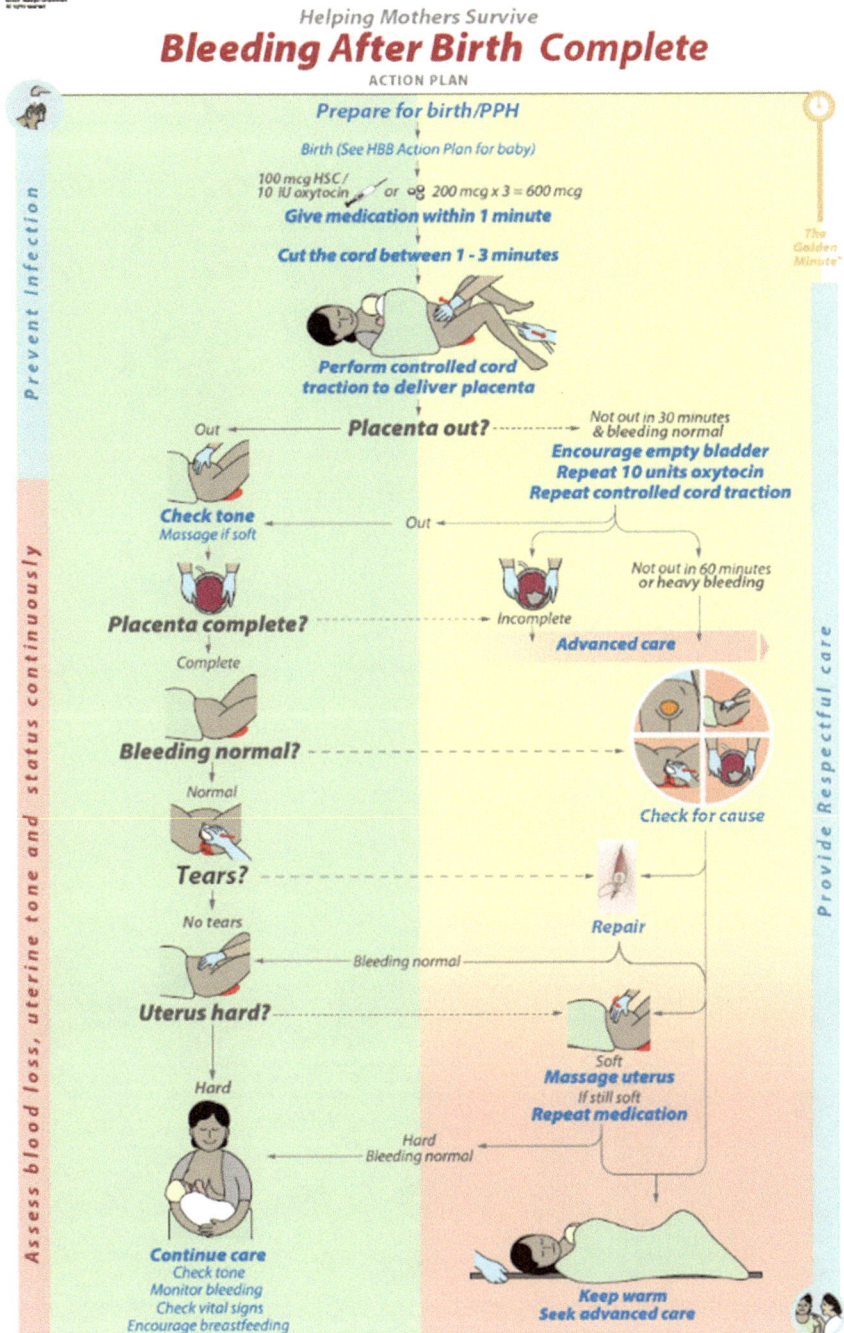

©2022 Jhpiego Corporation
All rights reserved

Helping Mothers Survive

Bleeding After Birth Complete

ACTION PLAN

Prepare for birth/PPH

Birth (See HBB Action Plan for baby)

100 mcg HSC /
10 IU oxytocin   or   200 mcg x 3 = 600 mcg
Give medication within 1 minute

Cut the cord between 1 - 3 minutes

**Perform controlled cord
traction to deliver placenta**

Out ◄──────── **Placenta out?** ┄┄┄► Not out in 30 minutes
& bleeding normal
**Encourage empty bladder
Repeat 10 units oxytocin
Repeat controlled cord traction**

Check tone
Massage if soft   Out ◄

Placenta complete? ┄┄► *Incomplete*   Not out in 60 minutes
or heavy bleeding

Complete   **Advanced care**

Bleeding normal? ┄┄┄┄┄

Normal   **Check for cause**

Tears?

No tears   *Repair*

Uterus hard? ┄┄┄┄   *Bleeding normal* ◄────

Soft
Massage uterus
If still soft
Repeat medication

Hard   *Hard
Bleeding normal*

Continue care
*Check tone
Monitor bleeding
Check vital signs
Encourage breastfeeding*   **Keep warm
Seek advanced care**

Prevent Infection

Assess blood loss, uterine tone and status continuously

Provide Respectful care

The Golden Minute"

Fig. 4.12 After birth action plan bleeding after birth and manage PPH + refractory care 'draft-version'. (Developed by Jhpiego, an affiliate of Johns Hopkins University, in collaboration with global partners and with graphic design support from Laerdal Global health)

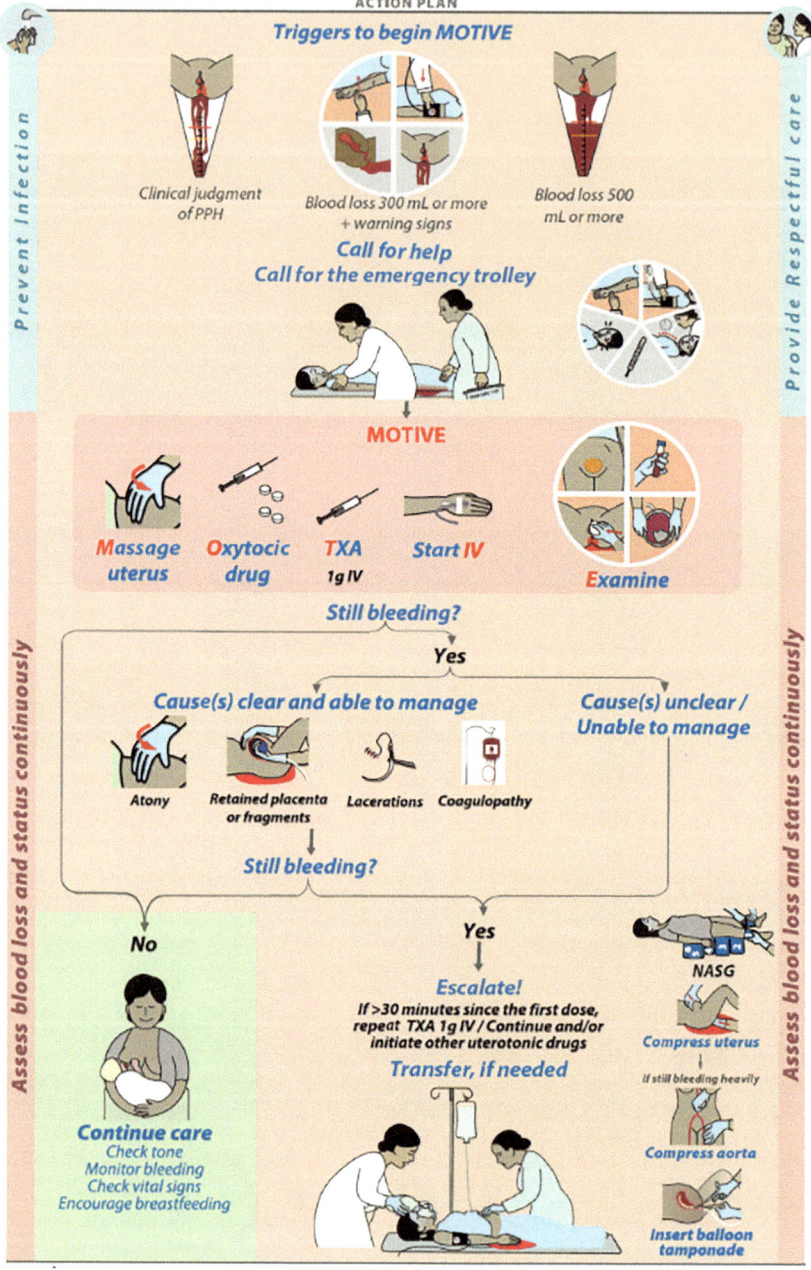

Fig. 4.13 Action plan bleeding after birth and manage PPH refractory care 'draft-version'. (Developed by Jhpiego, an affiliate of Johns Hopkins University, in collaboration with global partners and with graphic design support from Laerdal Global health)

Fig. 4.14 Nonpneumatic antishock garment

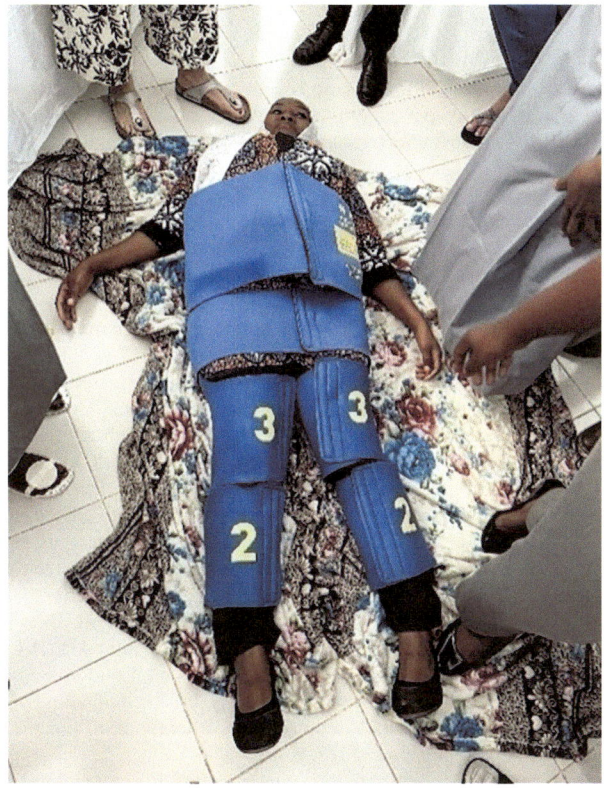

4.4 Prevention

Beside the active management of the third stage of labour improvement, an early detection of PPH was recently published for vaginal deliveries [14]. The first-line treatments for PPH (uterus massage, oxytocin IV, tranexamic acid iv, crystalloid fluids, and evaluation for escalation) were immediately administered when triggered by a blood loss of 300 mL or more if there was an accompanying abnormality in the vital signs or clinical observation. Blood loss was measured by a calibrated blood collection drape.

4.5 Conclusion

Management of PPH requires the coordinated action of a well-prepared team. Preventing haemorrhage by active management of the third stage of labour, recognizing haemorrhage in a timely manner, and calling for help early as well as structured stepwise actions following an algorithm are all essential steps to reduce morbidity and mortality from PPH.

References

1. https://www.glowm.com/resource-type/resource/textbook/title/a-/title/a-comprehensive-textbook-of-postpartum-hemorrhage-2nd-edition/resource-doc/1275.
2. WHO. WHO recommendations for the prevention and treatment of postpartum haemorrhage. 2012.
3. Begley CM, Gyte GM, Devane D, McGuire W, Weeks A, Biesty LM. Active versus expectant management for women in the third stage of labour. Cochrane Database Syst Rev. 2019;2(2):CD007412.
4. Queensland Health. Queensland Clinical Guidelines postpartum haemorrhage Guideline No. MN18.1V10-R23. 2021.
5. The PROMPT Editorial Team. PROMPT course manual, practical obstetric multi-professional training. 3rd ed. Cambridge University Press; 2017.
6. Knight M, Bunch K, Felker A, Patel R, Kotnis R, Kenyon S, Kurinczuk JJ. Saving lives, improving mothers' care. MBRRACE-UK; 2023.
7. https://globalhealthmedia.org/videos/uterine-balloon-tamponade/.
8. Dueckelmann AM, Hinkson L, Nonnenmacher A, Siedentopf JP, Schoenborn I, Weizsaecker K, et al. Uterine packing with chitosan-covered gauze compared to balloon tamponade for managing postpartum hemorrhage. Eur J Obstet Gynecol Reprod Biol. 2019;240:151–5.
9. B-Lynch C, Shah H. Conservative surgical management. In: Arulkumaran S, Karoshi M, Keith LG, Lalonde AB, B-Lynch C, editors. A comprehensive textbook of postpartum hemorrhage. 2nd ed. London: Sapiens Publishing; 2012. p. 433–40.
10. B-Lynch C, Keith LG, Campbell WB. Internal Iliac (hypogastric) artery ligation. In: Arulkumaran S, Karoshi M, Keith LG, Lalonde AB, B-Lynch C, editors. A comprehensive textbook of postpartum hemorrhage. 2nd ed. London: Sapiens Publishing; 2012. p. 441–7.
11. Baskett TF. Peripartum hysterectomy. In: Arulkumaran S, Karoshi M, Keith LG, Lalonde AB, B-Lynch C, editors. A comprehensive textbook of postpartum hemorrhage. 2nd ed. London: Sapiens Publishing; 2012. p. 462–5.
12. https://oss-online.ca/knowledge-base/pph-hys/#technique-total-hysterectomy.
13. WHO Guidelines Approved by the Guidelines Review Committee. WHO recommendations on the assessment of postpartum blood loss and use of a treatment bundle for postpartum haemorrhage. Geneva: World Health Organization; 2023.
14. Gallos I, Devall A, Martin J, Middleton L, Beeson L, Galadanci H, et al. Randomized trial of early detection and treatment of postpartum hemorrhage. N Engl J Med. 2023;389(1):11–21.
15. Hoesli I, et al. B-Lynch-uterine suture with a model. 2020.

Open Access This chapter is licensed under the terms of the Creative Commons Attribution 4.0 International License (http://creativecommons.org/licenses/by/4.0/), which permits use, sharing, adaptation, distribution and reproduction in any medium or format, as long as you give appropriate credit to the original author(s) and the source, provide a link to the Creative Commons license and indicate if changes were made.

The images or other third party material in this chapter are included in the chapter's Creative Commons license, unless indicated otherwise in a credit line to the material. If material is not included in the chapter's Creative Commons license and your intended use is not permitted by statutory regulation or exceeds the permitted use, you will need to obtain permission directly from the copyright holder.

Chapter 5
Uterine Inversion

5.1 Introduction: Background and Evidence

Key Learning Points
- Recognize uterine inversion and maternal shock accompanying it.
- Be able to perform the manual replacement technique.
- Understand that the placenta must be removed after uterus replacement.
- Be prepared to manage subsequent PPH.

Common Issues in the Management of Uterine Inversion [1]
- Difficulty and delay in recognizing the problem
- Delay in beginning resuscitation and manual replacement of the uterus
- Not being prepared to manage subsequent postpartum haemorrhage

Uterine inversion (Fig. 5.1) is a rare complication of childbirth, estimated to occur in 1/5000 to 1/20,000 births. The definition and risk factors are presented in Tables 5.1 and 5.2, respectively.

Supplementary Information The online version contains supplementary material available at https://doi.org/10.1007/978-3-031-81931-5_5.

© The Author(s) 2025, corrected publication 2025
C. Monod et al., *Simulation Training for Obstetric Emergencies in Low-Resource Countries*, https://doi.org/10.1007/978-3-031-81931-5_5

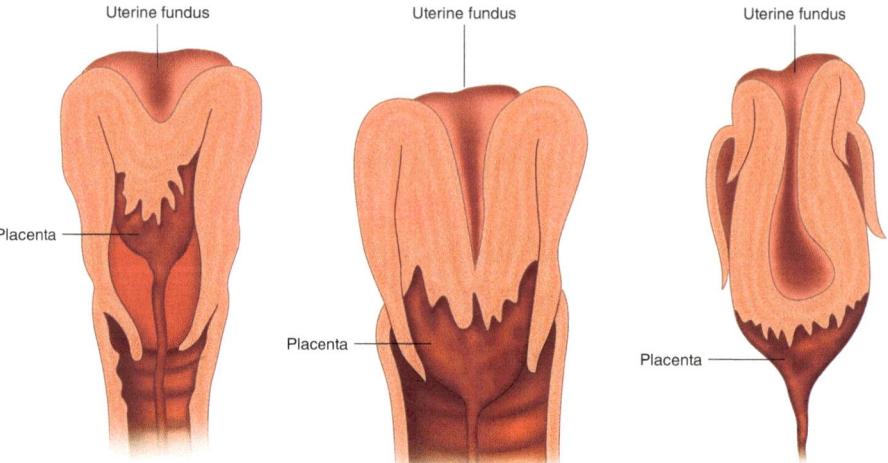

Fig. 5.1 Uterine inversion

Table 5.1 Definition of uterine inversion [2]

Uterine inversion
The fundus of the uterus descends through the genital tract, turning the uterus inside out

Table 5.2 Risk factors for uterine inversion [2]

Risks factors for uterine inversion
Too strong traction of the umbilical cord in the third stage of labour
Adherent placenta
Excessive fundal pressure
Multiparity
Very rapid birth
Macrosomia

5.2 Management

5.2.1 Diagnosis

Recognizing uterine inversion may be challenging when the uterine fundus does not appear at the introitus. The most common first sign is a sudden maternal shock with minimal vaginal bleeding. Typically, the woman may show bradycardia due to parasympathetic nerves stimulation. Consider uterine inversion when the uterus is not well palpable from the abdomen and perform a vaginal examination to make the

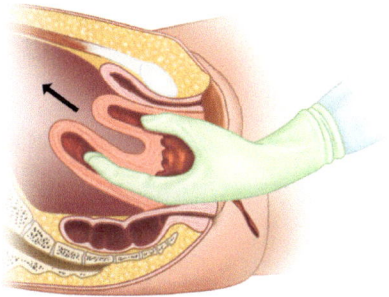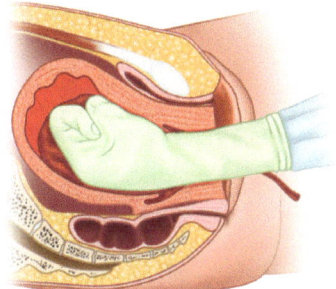

Fig. 5.2 Manual reposition of an inverted uterus

diagnosis. The most effective way to treat maternal shock is to replace the uterus (Fig. 5.2). Remove the placenta only AFTER you have replaced the uterus. Up to 90% of women develop atonic postpartum haemorrhage after uterine inversion. Be prepared to manage it!

- Call for help.
- Give oxygen.

- Manage maternal shock as described in Chap. 4 (PPH) and replace the uterus simultaneously.

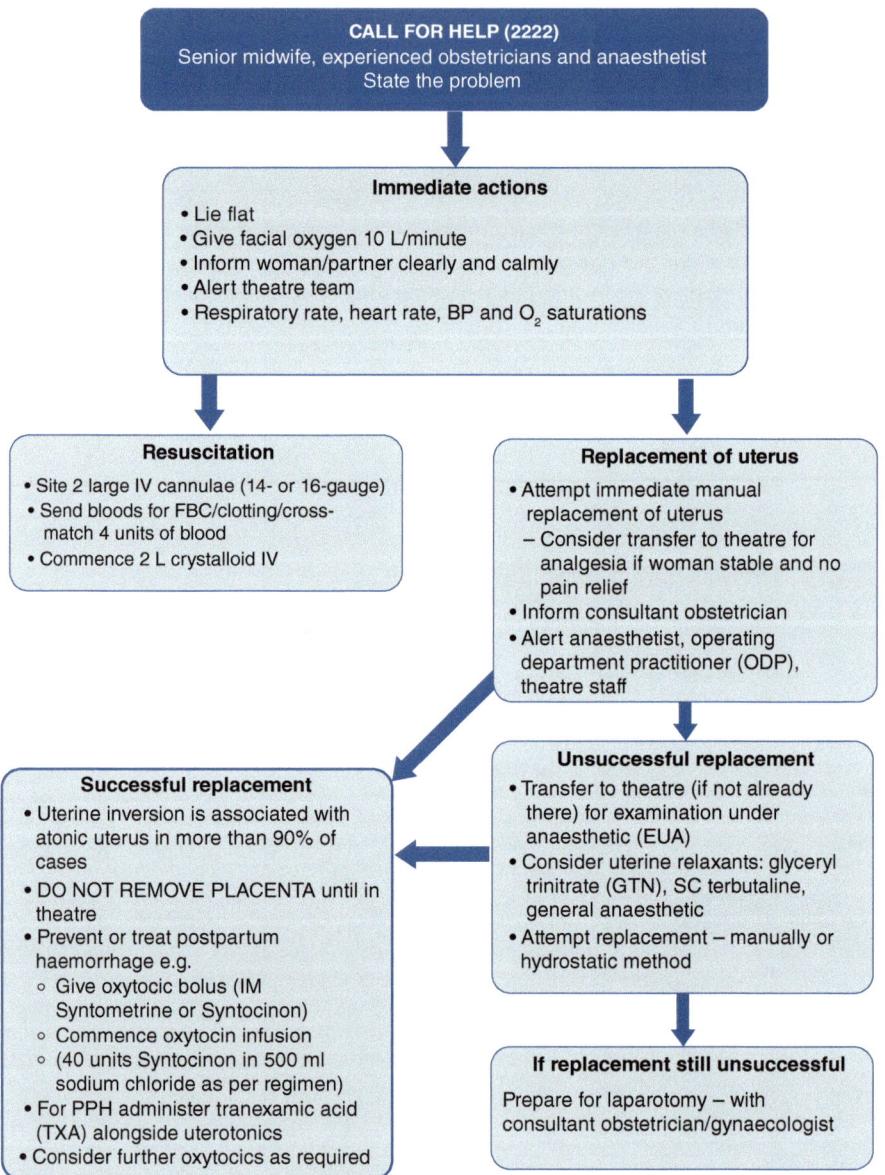

Fig. 5.3 Uterine inversion algorithm [2]. (Reproduced with permission of the Licensor Through PLSclear)

5.3 Algorithm

Figure 5.3 depicts the management algorithm of uterine inversion.

5.4 Conclusion

Uterine inversion is a rare complication of childbirth that may be challenging to recognize. Replace the uterus quickly and manage the postpartum haemorrhage.

References

1. Burns R, Dent K. Managing medical and obstetric emergencies and trauma. The MOET course manual. 4th ed. Cambridge University Press; 2022.
2. The PROMPT Editorial Team. PROMPT course manual, practical obstetric multi-professional training. 3rd ed. Cambridge University Press; 2017.
3. youTube. Uterine inversion_obstetric podcast. Uterine inversion. 2018. https://www.youtube.com/watch?v=bYIPkNfPDUI&t=4s.

Open Access This chapter is licensed under the terms of the Creative Commons Attribution 4.0 International License (http://creativecommons.org/licenses/by/4.0/), which permits use, sharing, adaptation, distribution and reproduction in any medium or format, as long as you give appropriate credit to the original author(s) and the source, provide a link to the Creative Commons license and indicate if changes were made.

The images or other third party material in this chapter are included in the chapter's Creative Commons license, unless indicated otherwise in a credit line to the material. If material is not included in the chapter's Creative Commons license and your intended use is not permitted by statutory regulation or exceeds the permitted use, you will need to obtain permission directly from the copyright holder.

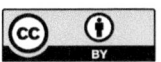

Chapter 6
Antepartum Haemorrhage

6.1 Introduction: Background and Evidence

Antepartum haemorrhage (APH) is often unpredictable and can endanger the life of pregnant woman and her foetus. Marginal placental bleeding is a common cause of minor APH, whereas placenta praevia and placental abruption (Fig. 6.1) are commonly responsible of major APH. Uterine rupture, during labour but also after trauma such as road traffic accidents, also leads to major APH. Bleeding from a vasa praevia, a foetal vessel lying just over the cervical ostium, can also cause APH. Even when the amount of vaginal bleeding is limited, this can lead to severe foetal anaemia and foetal death. Vasa praevia may be very difficult to identify, both on clinical examination and on ultrasound. In most situations, vaginal bleeding is obvious. However, APH (like PPH) can also be concealed intra-abdominally or within the uterus. In this case, symptoms and signs of shock/maternal collapse are the first presenting features. Table 6.1 presents common features of the different causes of APH.

© The Author(s) 2025
C. Monod et al., *Simulation Training for Obstetric Emergencies in Low-Resource Countries*, https://doi.org/10.1007/978-3-031-81931-5_6

Fig. 6.1 Placental
abruption

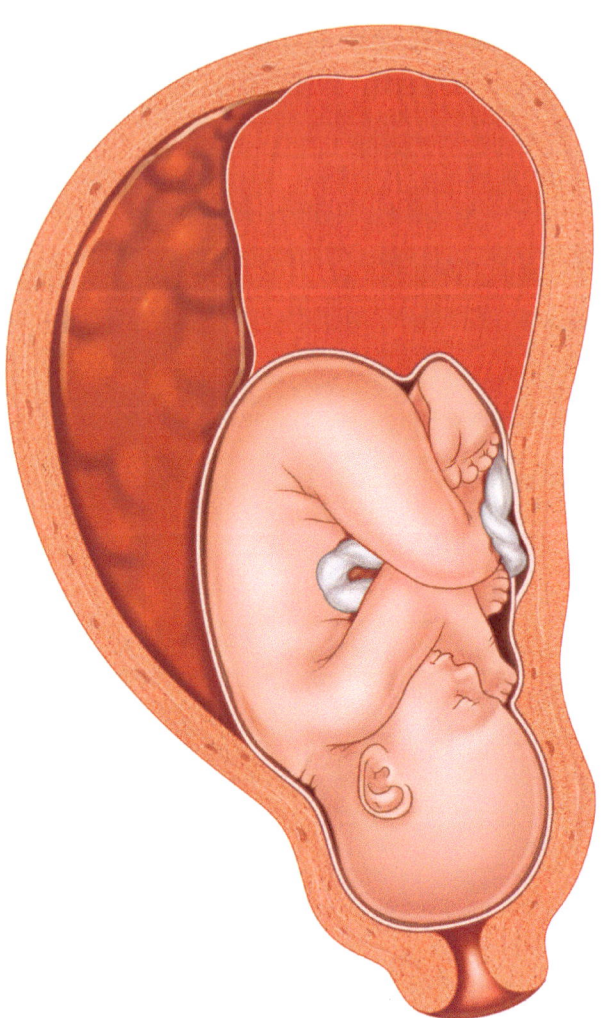

Table 6.1 Common feature of different causes of APH [1]

Cause	Possible presenting features	Condition of uterus	Condition of fetus	Risk factors/ contributory factors
Placenta praevia	• Painless vaginal bleeding • High presenting part or transverse lie • Shock	• Non-tender and soft or irritable uterus	• Depending on amount of blood loss	• Low-lying placenta on antenatal ultrasound • Previous uterine surgery, e.g. caesarean section • IVF
Placental abruption	• Bleeding (may be concealed) • Constant pain • Shock • Fetal compromise (abnormal/ pathological CTG)	• Tender, woody, hard uterus • Irritable uterus	• Depending on blood loss and timing since abruption occurred	• Previous abruption (up to 25% recurrence rate if two previous abruptions) • Pre-eclampsia/ hypertension • Fetal growth restriction • Cocaine use • Smoking • Abdominal trauma • Grand multiparity
Uterine rupture	• Sudden onset of constant sharp pain • Peritonism • Abnormal/ pathological CTG • Very high or unreachable presenting part • Bleeding (may be concealed) • Shock • Haematuria	• Contractions may cease	• Likely to have abnormal/ pathological CTG • Fetus palpable ex utero	• Previous uterine surgery (caesarean section, myomectomy, cornual/ectopic pregnancy) • Parity ≥4 • Trauma • Oxytocin infusion during labour
Vasa praevia	• Variable fresh PV blood loss after rupture of membranes • Acute fetal compromise • No maternal shock	• Normal	• Acute fetal compromise (sinusoidal/ bradycardic CTG) • Fetal mortality 33–100%	• Low-lying placenta • Succenturiate lobe

Reproduced with permission of the Licensor through PLSclear

6.2 Management

The management of APH requires the coordinated, simultaneous initiation of differ-ent actions. At the same time, an assessment of the condition of the woman, of the foetus, and of the cause of APH should be performed. The specific measures to be taken depend on the cause and the available resources. If the amount of blood loss compromises the condition of the pregnant woman, resuscitation measures and stopping the bleeding to save her life should have priority. In this situation, expedit-ing birth should not be delayed for foetal reasons (e.g. to administer steroids for foetal lung maturation) at any gestational age. If available, a paediatric team should be called to take care of the baby after birth, as it may need resuscitation measures or blood transfusion, too.

Figure 6.2 describes the general principles of evaluation and management of APH.

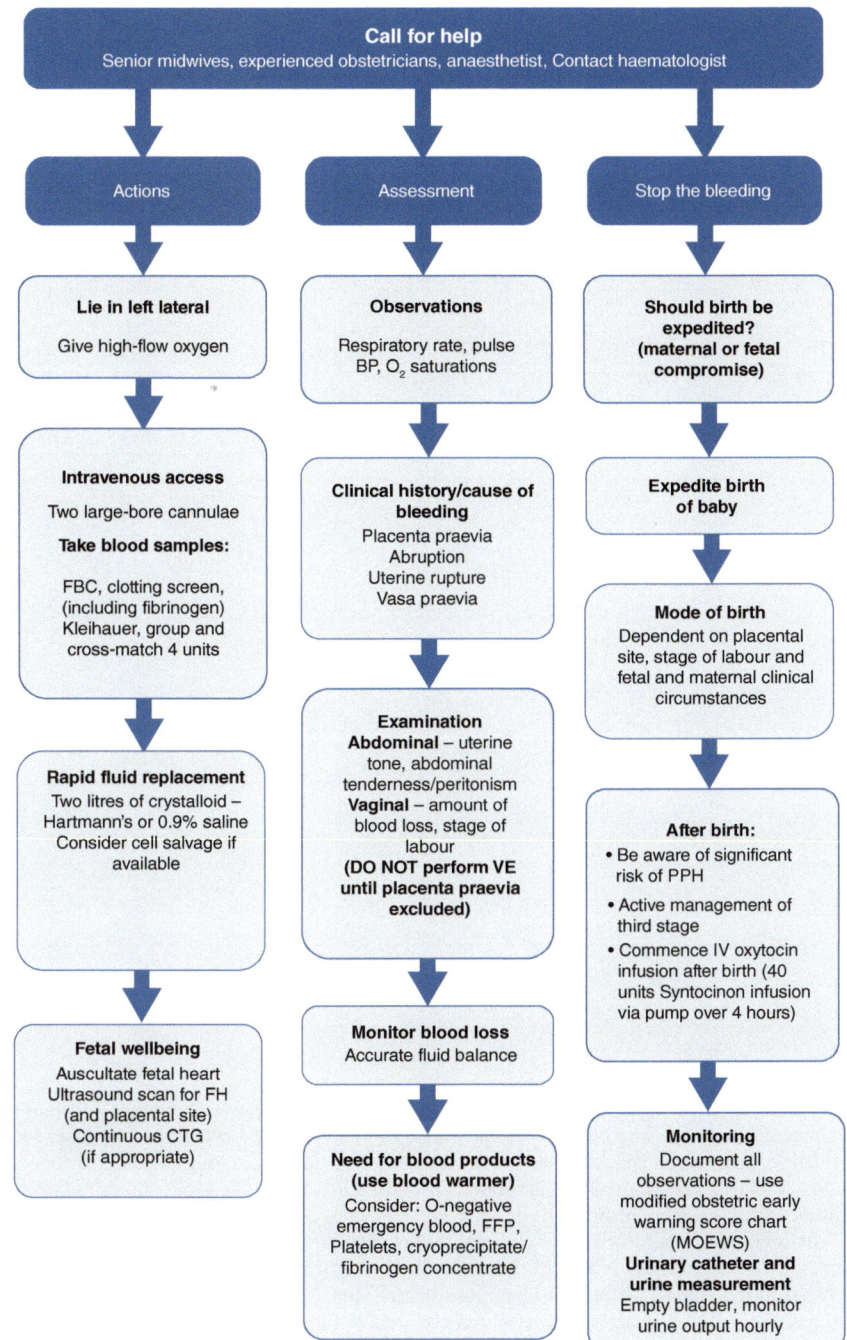

Fig. 6.2 Initial evaluation and management in APH [1]. (Reproduced with permission of the Licensor Through PLSclear)

6.3   Conclusion

APH is a complex symptom caused by different causes, from benign to life-threatening for the mother and the foetus. The decision to deliver can be particularly challenging.

Reference

1. The PROMPT Editorial Team. PROMPT course manual, practical obstetric multi-professional training. 3rd ed. Cambridge University Press; 2017.

Open Access   This chapter is licensed under the terms of the Creative Commons Attribution 4.0 International License (http://creativecommons.org/licenses/by/4.0/), which permits use, sharing, adaptation, distribution and reproduction in any medium or format, as long as you give appropriate credit to the original author(s) and the source, provide a link to the Creative Commons license and indicate if changes were made.

The images or other third party material in this chapter are included in the chapter's Creative Commons license, unless indicated otherwise in a credit line to the material. If material is not included in the chapter's Creative Commons license and your intended use is not permitted by statutory regulation or exceeds the permitted use, you will need to obtain permission directly from the copyright holder.

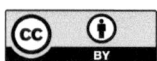

Chapter 7
Pre-eclampsia and Eclampsia

7.1 Introduction: Background and Evidence

Key Learning Points
- Recognise signs and symptoms of pre-eclampsia with severe features (severe pre-eclampsia).
- Understand the severity of complications of very high blood pressure (severe hypertension: systolic blood pressure ≥160 mmHg).
- Know how to treat severe hypertension.
- Manage eclamptic fit correctly and expeditiously.
- Know which surveillance to perform on a woman receiving IV magnesium sulphate.

Frequent Challenges
- Not stating the problem clearly
- Forgetting to call for help, particularly for an obstetrician and/or anaesthetist
- Inadequate treatment of severe hypertension (systolic blood pressure ≥160 mmHg)
- Failure to stabilize the woman before expediting birth
- Forgetting to perform basic resuscitation measures in case of eclamptic fits

Hypertensive disorders, pre-eclampsia, and eclampsia are the second most common cause of maternal death worldwide. Severe hypertension (systolic blood pressure ≥160 mmHg) greatly threatens the mother's health and life as well as the life of the foetus. Inadequate treatment may lead to maternal intracranial haemorrhage and subsequently to severe neurologic sequelae or even death. Neglecting to control hypertension represents a major failure in the care of women with pre-eclampsia or eclampsia.

Definitions
Tables 7.1, 7.2, 7.3, and 7.4 present the definitions of pre-eclampsia, eclampsia, and hypertension.

© The Author(s) 2025
C. Monod et al., *Simulation Training for Obstetric Emergencies in Low-Resource Countries*, https://doi.org/10.1007/978-3-031-81931-5_7

Table 7.1 Definition of hypertension chronic hypertension and gestational hypertension adapted from different international societies [10, 11]

Condition	Definition
Hypertension in pregnancy	Blood pressure ≥140 mmHg systolic or ≥90 mmHg diastolic or both
Severe hypertension in pregnancy	Blood pressure ≥160 mmHg systolic or ≥110 mmHg diastolic or both
Chronic hypertension	Blood pressure ≥140 mmHg systolic or ≥90 mmHg diastolic or both before pregnancy or before 20 weeks of pregnancy and does not resolve after pregnancy
Gestational hypertension	New hypertension presenting after 20 weeks of pregnancy without significant proteinuria

Table 7.2 WHO definition of pre-eclampsia [1]

Condition	Diagnostic criteria
Pre-eclampsia	Onset of a new episode of hypertension during pregnancy, characterized by • Persistent hypertension (diastolic blood pressure ≥90 mmHg) and • **Substantial proteinuria (>300mg/24 h; urine dipstick testing protein 2+ or 3+)**
Eclampsia	Generalized seizure, generally in addition to pre-eclampsia criteria

Table 7.3 New definition of pre-eclampsia adapted from different international societies [2, 10, 12]

Pre-eclampsia
New onset of hypertension (blood pressure ≥140 mmHg systolic or ≥90 mmHg diastolic) on two occasions 4 h apart after 20 weeks of pregnancy and the coexistence of one or more of the following new-onset conditions:
• Proteinuria (≥300 mg/24 h or protein/creatinine ratio ≥30 mg/mmol or 2+ on dipstick testing) **or**

• Other maternal organ dysfunction:
  – Renal insufficiency (creatinine ≥0.9 mg/dL)
  – Liver involvement (liver enzymes elevated to twice the normal concentration or more, with or without right upper quadrant or epigastric abdominal pain)
  – Neurological complications such as eclampsia, altered mental status, blindness, stroke, clonus, severe headaches, or persistent visual scotoma
  – Pulmonary oedema
  – Haematological complications such as thrombocytopenia (platelet count below 100,000/µL), disseminated intravascular coagulation, or haemolysis

• Signs of placental dysfunction such as intrauterine growth retardation (small baby) and stillbirth

Table 7.4 Definition of pre-eclampsia with severe features adapted from different international societies [2, 10, 12]

Severe (imminent) pre-eclampsia
Pre-eclampsia with severe hypertension that does not respond to treatment or is associated with
• Ongoing or recurring severe headaches
• Visual disturbance (blurring, flashing, scotoma)
• Nausea or vomiting
• Epigastric pain
• Oliguria
• Progressive deterioration in laboratory blood tests such as rising creatinine or liver transaminases or falling platelet count

Table 7.5 Risk factors for pre-eclampsia adapted from [5]

Risk factors for pre-eclampsia
Nulliparity or interval >10 years since last pregnancy
History of (pre-)eclampsia in a previous pregnancy
Chronic hypertension
Family history of pre-eclampsia
Diabetes
Multiple pregnancy
Obesity
Extreme maternal ages (<18 or >40 years old)
Renal disease

The WHO definition of pre-eclampsia is based on diastolic hypertension and presence of proteinuria. However, in a non-negligible number of cases, pre-eclampsia or eclampsia evolves in an atypical and fulminant way, where proteinuria does not appear or appears only at a later point. Therefore, newer definitions do not require proteinuria to diagnose pre-eclampsia or eclampsia. Hypertension associated with at least one maternal organ dysfunction is sufficient to diagnose it. In addition, it is important to consider systolic hypertension, too. High systolic blood pressure is the primary determinant of maternal intracranial complications such as intracranial haemorrhage. This was not considered in the older definitions of pre-eclampsia. New definitions of pre-eclampsia replace the term "severe pre-eclampsia" with "pre-eclampsia with severe features" to emphasise that pre-eclampsia does not progress from mild to severe in a straight line. In most cases, the progression of the disease and the development of severe features is unpredictable and women should be monitored closely at all stages of the disease [12].

Several risk factors (Table 7.5) predispose a pregnant woman to develop pre-eclampsia, but the disease may occur in any pregnant woman.

Eclamptic Fit
Eclampsia presents with generalized seizures—jerking limb and head movements. Cyanosis, tongue biting, and loss of urine may also occur. In most cases, eclamptic

Table 7.6 Maternal complications of pre-eclampsia adapted from [5]

Maternal complications of pre-eclampsia
Intracranial haemorrhage (leading cause of death from pre-eclampsia/eclampsia)
Placental abruption
Eclampsia
HELLP syndrome (**h**aemolysis, **e**levated **l**iver enzymes, **l**ow **p**latelets)
Disseminated intravascular coagulation
Renal failure
Pulmonary oedema
Acute respiratory distress syndrome (ARDS)

Table 7.7 Foetal complications of pre-eclampsia adapted from [5]

Foetal complications of pre-eclampsia
Foetal growth restriction (small baby)
Hypoxia
Placental abruption
Medically indicated preterm birth

Table 7.8 Symptoms and signs of pre-eclampsia

Symptoms and signs of pre-eclampsia
Headache
Visual disturbances
Vomiting
Epigastric or right upper abdominal quadrant tenderness or pain
Hyperreflexia with/without clonus
Oedema (especially facial) or pulmonary oedema
Recently developed high blood pressure
Proteinuria
Rapidly deteriorating haematological and biochemical parameters in blood test

fits are self-limiting and last for <90 s. Mothers with eclampsia frequently experience severe associated morbidities (as described in Table 7.6). The child also has a high risk of perinatal mortality (Table 7.7).

In pre-eclampsia, the placenta is not functioning properly, a condition called 'placental insufficiency', which leads to several foetal and neonatal complications as described in Table 7.7.

Pre-eclampsia is a multisystem disorder. The presenting symptoms and signs reflect this fact. Symptoms and signs that should raise concern that the woman may have pre-eclampsia are described in Table 7.8.

7.2   Management of Pre-eclampsia with Severe Features and Eclampsia

7.2.1   Initial Management of Pre-eclampsia with Severe Features and Eclampsia

Initial management of eclampsia includes basic supportive measures, control of seizures, and prevention of their recurrence with magnesium sulphate, preferably intravenously (Fig. 7.1). The initial assessment and management of pre-eclampsia with

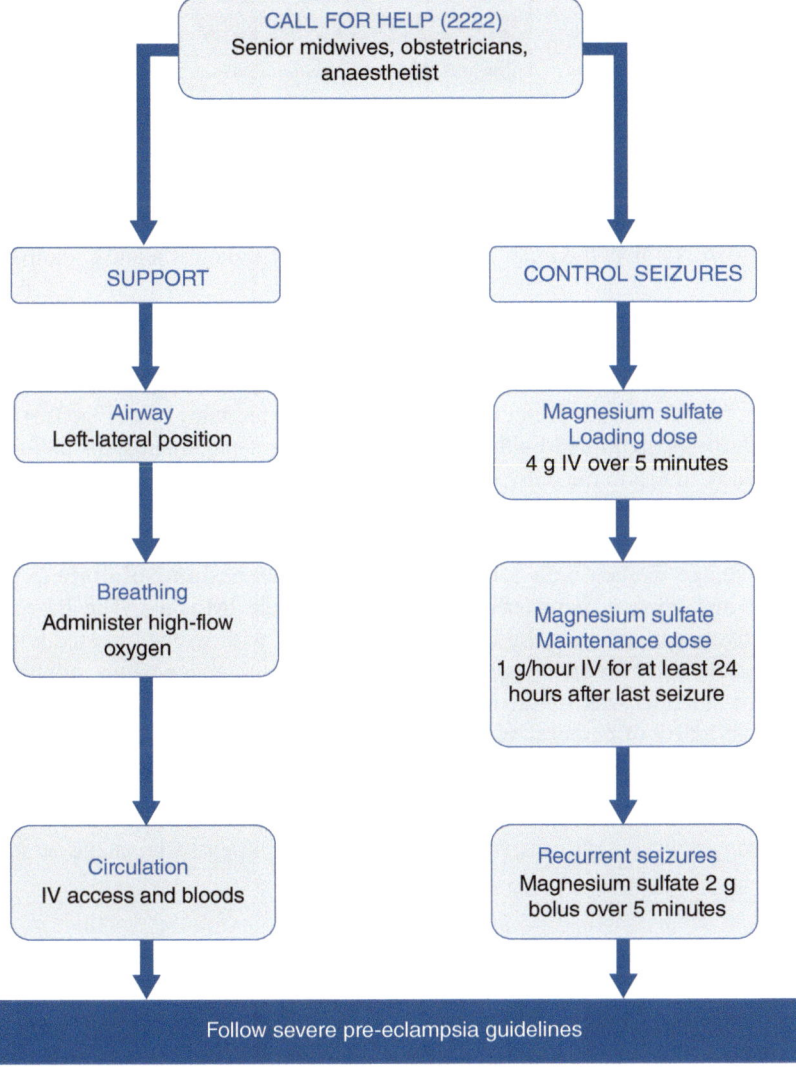

Fig. 7.1 Initial management of pre-eclampsia with severe features (severe pre-eclampsia)/eclampsia [5]. (Reproduced with permission of the Licensor Through PLSclear)

Fig. 7.2 Magnesium regimen in pre-eclampsia and eclampsia [3]. (Copyright 2024 with permission from Elsevier)

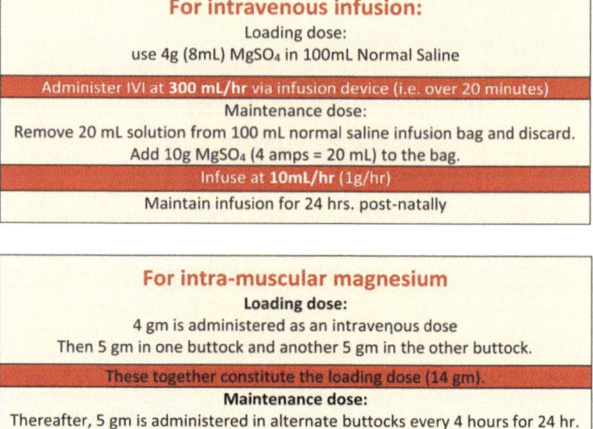

severe features (severe pre-eclampsia) are essentially the same. Although no seizures have occurred in pre-eclampsia with severe features (severe pre-eclampsia) yet, administer magnesium sulphate to prevent them.

Figure 7.2 depicts the magnesium regimen in pre-eclampsia and eclampsia [3].

7.2.1.1 Emergency Box 'Pre-eclampsia/Eclampsia'

It is beneficial to have a pre-eclampsia/eclampsia emergency box (Fig. 7.3) with all material, drugs, and local guidelines depicting the management steps and doses of drugs ready to use in the delivery room or emergency department. It saves precious time when managing a woman with these conditions and helps the team stay calm and organized.

To manage women with eclampsia, use only **magnesium sulphate** to manage seizures and prevent recurrence. Prefer the IV to the IM route. The IV route has fewer adverse effects than the IM route. Compared with women treated with other drugs, such as benzodiazepines, women treated with magnesium sulphate have recurrent seizures less frequently. Magnesium sulphate is thought to reverse the vasoconstriction of cerebral vessels. Remember that the first seizure is often self-limiting. **Magnesium sulphate prevents the recurrence of seizures**.

> In women with eclampsia, use only magnesium sulphate to manage seizures.

7.2.1.2 Magnesium Sulphate Toxicity

The kidneys extract magnesium sulphate. If the urine output is normal, there is little risk that a woman under a routine magnesium sulphate regimen will suffer magnesium toxicity. However, if the woman becomes oliguric (urine output <100 mL over

Fig. 7.3 Emergency box for pre-eclampsia/eclampsia

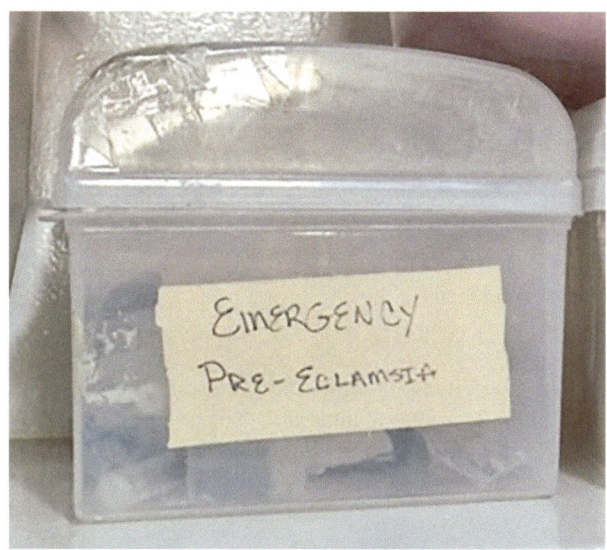

Fig. 7.4 Symptoms and signs of magnesium sulphate toxicity. (Adapted from [5])

Loss of deep tendon reflexes (patelar reflexes)

Respiratory depression

Respiratory arrest

Cardiac arrest

Table 7.9 Actions in case of magnesium sulphate toxicity adapted from [5]

Cardiopulmonary arrest on magnesium sulphate
Stop magnesium sulphate infusion
Start maternal resuscitation
Administer 10% calcium gluconate 10 mL IV in 10 min
Continue reanimation manoeuvres until breathing resumes

4 h), the risk of toxicity increases. In these circumstances, administrating only the loading dose of magnesium sulphate on admission can be an option. The infusion should be stopped if the woman is already on a maintenance dose. In the situation of diminished urine output, magnesium sulphate levels should be determined in the blood (therapeutic range 2–4 mmol/L). Symptoms and signs of magnesium sulphate toxicity, as well as the emergency actions in case of magnesium sulphate intoxication, are illustrated in Fig. 7.4 and Table 7.9).

7.2.2 Control High Blood Pressure (Hypertension)

Lowering high blood pressure can be lifesaving. Therefore, treating hypertension promptly and effectively is essential. Hypertension puts the woman at risk of intracranial haemorrhage, neurological sequelae, and death. Systolic hypertension represents the most significant risk of intracranial haemorrhage (Fig. 7.5) [12].

Blood pressure target in pre-eclampsia/eclampsia
Systolic:135 mmHg
Diastolic: 85 mmHg

Most guidelines recommend oral nifedipine, alpha methyldopa, beta blockers including parenteral labetalol, or parenteral hydralazine. Therefore, these agents would seem to be reasonable choices [4, 6, 7, 12].

Severe Hypertension

Manifestation: Systolic BP ≥160 mm Hg or diastolic BP ≥110 mm Hg
Objective: Systolic BP <160 mm Hg and diastolic BP <110 mm Hg within 180 min
Management: Choose one of the following four classes of drugs and the preferred route and timing of administration
   If BP control is not achieved despite maximal doses, move to another class of medication
   If BP control is not achieved by 360 min despite 2 medications, consult critical care, consider ICU admission, stabilize and
      deliver (if undelivered)

First-Line Drug	Route of Administration and Dosage Units	0 Min	30 Min	60 Min	90 Min	120 Min	150 Min
Labetalol	Oral — mg	200	—	200	—	200	—
	Intermittent IV — mg	10–20	20–40	40–80	40–80	40–80	40–80
	IV infusion — mg/min	0.5–2.0	→	→	→	→	→
Nifedipine	Oral capsule — mg	5–10	10	—	10	—	10
	Oral tablet (PA/MR) — mg	10	—	10	—	10	—
Hydralazine	Intermittent IV — mg	5	5–10	5–10	5–10	—	—
Methyldopa	Oral (if other medications unavailable or for in utero transfer without monitoring) — mg	1000	—	—	—	—	—

Fig. 7.5 Treatment of severe hypertension [7]. (Copyright © 2024, Massachusetts Medical Society. Reprinted with permission from Massachusetts Medical Society)

7.2.3 *Monitor*

The woman should be monitored regularly, as her condition may deteriorate rapidly. Observations should be documented accurately.

- Blood pressure, pulse, and respiratory rate should be taken every 15 min until stabilized, then every 30 min.
- A urine catheter should be inserted, and hourly urine output monitored.
- Hourly oxygen saturation should be monitored.
- A blood sample should be taken every 6–24 h (if available: full blood count, clotting screen, urea, urate, creatinine, electrolytes, and liver function tests).

If under magnesium sulphate, additionally check:

- Hourly deep tendon reflexes (patellar reflexes)
- Hourly respiratory rate

STOP Magnesium Sulphate if

- There is a loss of reflexes. When reflexes return, recommence infusion at 0.5 g/h.
- Oliguria is present (urine output <100 mL/4 h).
- Respiratory rate is <16 breaths/min.
- Oxygen saturation is <90%.

7.2.3.1 Monitoring of Fluid Balance and Prevention of Pulmonary Oedema

Women with pre-eclampsia with severe features (severe pre-eclampsia) or eclampsia are at risk of developing pulmonary oedema. It is defined as fluid accumulation in the lungs due to fluid overload and may lead to respiratory failure. Therefore, monitoring fluid intake and urine output is very important. The overall fluid intake (including all drugs administered intravenously, oral fluid intake, and infusions) should not exceed 1 mL/kg/h (about 80 mL/h). Symptoms and signs of pulmonary oedema are described in Table 7.10 and Fig. 7.6.

Table 7.10 Symptoms and signs of pulmonary oedema adapted from [5]

Symptoms and signs of pulmonary oedema	
Shortness of breath	Tachypnoea (high respiratory rate)
Inability to lie flat	Tachycardia (high pulse)
Inability to speak in full sentences	Crepitation at lung base (auscultation)
Confusion and agitation	Decreasing oxygen saturation
	Positive fluid balance (fluid overload)
	Frothy sputum

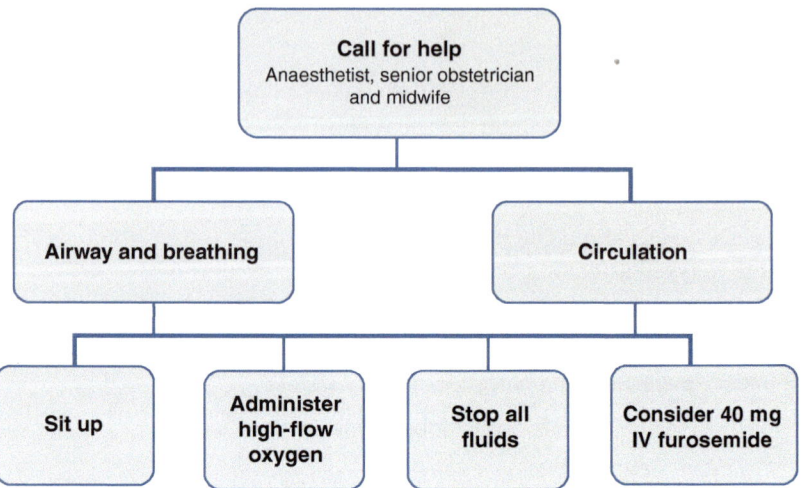

Fig. 7.6 Management of pulmonary oedema [5]. (Reproduced with permission of the Licensor Through PLSclear)

7.2.4   Make Plans for Birth [8]

Stabilize the woman before making plans for birth!

The only definitive treatment of pre-eclampsia/eclampsia is the baby's birth. Before planning for birth, the woman should be stabilized with magnesium sulphate and drugs to lower blood pressure. The decision to induce labour or perform a caesarean section is made on an individual basis, taking into consideration gestational age, severity or progression of pre-eclampsia, and condition of the woman. After an eclamptic fit, stabilize the woman and expedite the birth. If the pregnancy is less than 34 weeks, you should additionally discuss foetal lung maturation. There is general agreement that birth should be the aim if the woman has reached 37 weeks. Before 34–36 weeks, the benefit of expectant management for the foetus should be balanced with the risk to the woman. Before 34 weeks, the decision is even more challenging. If the foetus has reached viability and the woman is stable enough to postpone the birth for 48 h, then you should perform foetal lung maturation with corticosteroids as per local protocol. If the woman's state deteriorates before the 48 h, deliver the baby to protect the mother's life.

7.2.5 After Birth

Magnesium sulphate infusion should be continued for at least 24 h after birth. Worsening of the woman's condition and eclamptic fits can occur after birth. Therefore, you should continue regular monitoring after birth until the woman is entirely stable.

7.2.6 Transfer

If a woman with pre-eclampsia or eclampsia presents to a community care facility, she should be transferred to the next available hospital as soon as possible. Initial evaluation, prevention of seizure with magnesium sulphate, and control of blood pressure should occur before transferring the woman and all actions should be carefully documented for the transfer.

7.3 Algorithm

The algorithm for managing pre-eclampsia and eclampsia is shown in Fig. 7.7.

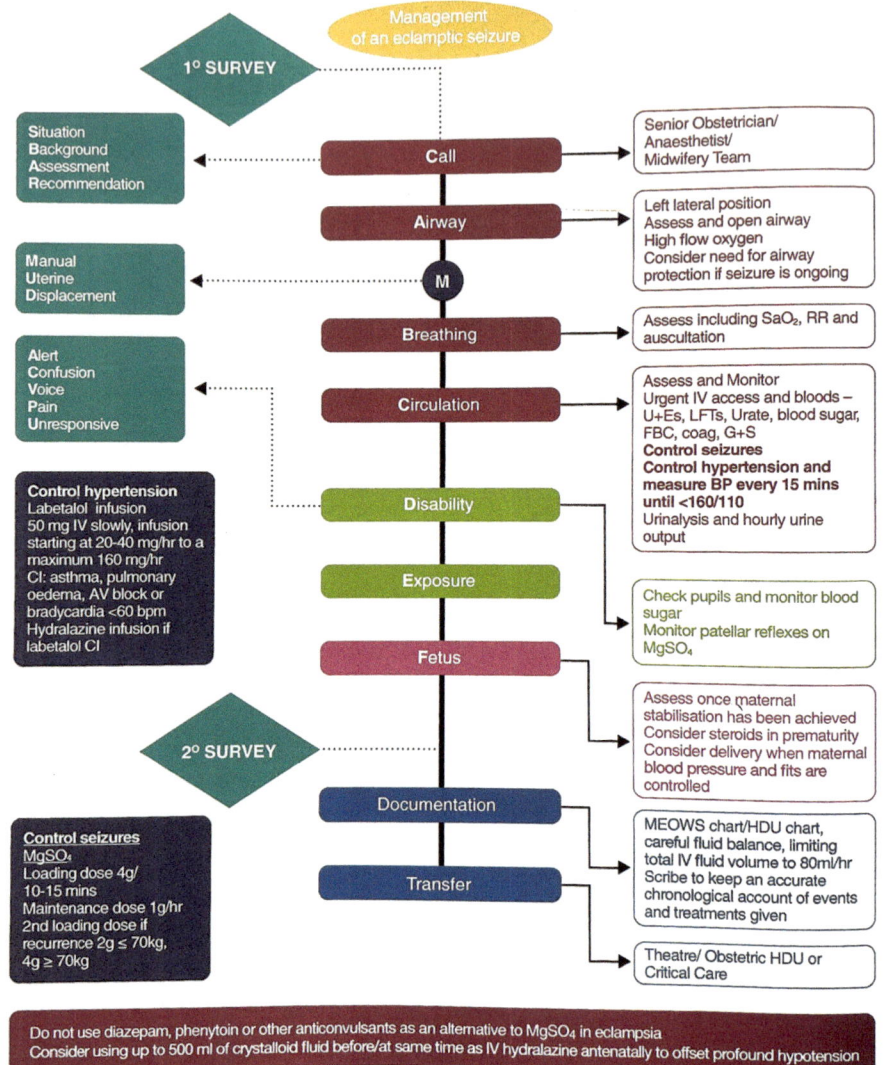

Fig. 7.7 Management of pre-eclampsia and eclampsia [9]. (Reproduced with permission of the Licensor Through PLSclear)

7.4 Conclusion

Control of high blood pressure and preventing recurrent seizures with magnesium sulphate as well as timely birth of the baby can be lifesaving for the pregnant woman and prevent severe neurological morbidity.

References

1. World Health Organization. WHO recommendations for prevention and treatment of pre-eclampsia and eclampsia. WHO; 2011.
2. Gestational hypertension and preeclampsia: ACOG Practice Bulletin, Number 222. Obstet Gynecol. 2020;135(6):e237–60.
3. Magee LA, Brown MA, Kenny LC, Karumanchi SA, Mc Carthy FP, Saito S et al. The hypertensive disorders of pregnancy: ISSHP classification, diagnosis & management recommendations for international practice. Pregnancy Hypertens. 2018;13:291–310.
4. World Health Organization. WHO recommendations: drug treatment for severe hypertension in pregnancy. WHO; 2018.
5. The PROMPT Editorial Team. PROMPT course manual, practical obstetric multi-professional training. 3rd ed. Cambridge University Press; 2017.
6. WHO. WHO essential medication list 2021. WHO; 2021.
7. Magee LA, Nicolaides KH, von Dadelszen P. Preeclampsia. N Engl J Med. 2022;386(19):1817–32.
8. World Health Organisation. WHO recommendations, policy of interventionist versus expectant management in severe pre-eclampsia before term. WHO; 2018.
9. Burns R, Dent K. Managing medical and obstetric emergencies and trauma. The MOET course manual. 4th ed. Cambridge University Press; 2022.
10. NICE Guideline. Hypertension in pregnancy: diagnosis and management. NICE; 2019.
11. American College of Obstetricians and Gynecologists' Committee on Practice Bulletins—Obstetrics. ACOG Practice Bulletin No. 203: Chronic hypertension in pregnancy. Obstet Gynecol. 2019;133(1):e26–50.
12. Magee LA, Brown MA, Hall DR, Gupte S, Hennessy A, Karumanchi SA, Kenny LC, McCarthy F, Myers J, Poon LC, Rana S, Saito S, Staff AC, Tsigas E, von Dadelszen P. The 2021 International Society for the Study of Hypertension in Pregnancy classification, diagnosis & management recommendations for international practice. Pregnancy Hypertens. 2022;27:148–169. https://doi.org/10.1016/j.preghy.2021.09.008.

Open Access This chapter is licensed under the terms of the Creative Commons Attribution 4.0 International License (http://creativecommons.org/licenses/by/4.0/), which permits use, sharing, adaptation, distribution and reproduction in any medium or format, as long as you give appropriate credit to the original author(s) and the source, provide a link to the Creative Commons license and indicate if changes were made.

The images or other third party material in this chapter are included in the chapter's Creative Commons license, unless indicated otherwise in a credit line to the material. If material is not included in the chapter's Creative Commons license and your intended use is not permitted by statutory regulation or exceeds the permitted use, you will need to obtain permission directly from the copyright holder.

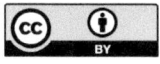

Chapter 8
Maternal Sepsis

8.1 Introduction: Background and Evidence

Key Learning Points
- Recognize maternal sepsis.
- Understand the need for early IV antibiotics and fluids.
- Know the steps in the emergency management of sepsis and septic shock.

Maternal sepsis (Fig. 8.1), a severe infection in pregnancy or after birth, is the third leading cause of maternal death worldwide, after postpartum haemorrhage and hypertensive disorders [1]. The new WHO 2016 definition of maternal sepsis is presented in Table 8.1.

8.1.1 Management

8.1.1.1 Sepsis Recognition

Time to treatment is essential to improve outcomes in sepsis. Early recognition is therefore crucial. However, recognizing sepsis may be very challenging, as symptoms are often unspecific. A pregnant woman or a woman who gave birth or had an abortion or miscarriage in the last 6 weeks is at higher risk of infection than other healthy adults (Fig. 8.2).

A woman should be suspected of having sepsis if she

- Looks unwell.
- Looks confused.
- Has a high or low temperature.
- Has low blood pressure and/or increased heart rate.
- Has decreased urine output.
- Is breathing fast.

© The Author(s) 2025
C. Monod et al., *Simulation Training for Obstetric Emergencies in Low-Resource Countries*, https://doi.org/10.1007/978-3-031-81931-5_8

Fig. 8.1 Maternal sepsis definition and management. (Reproduced from: WHO 2016 maternal sepsis definition and management [2], Copyright 2024)

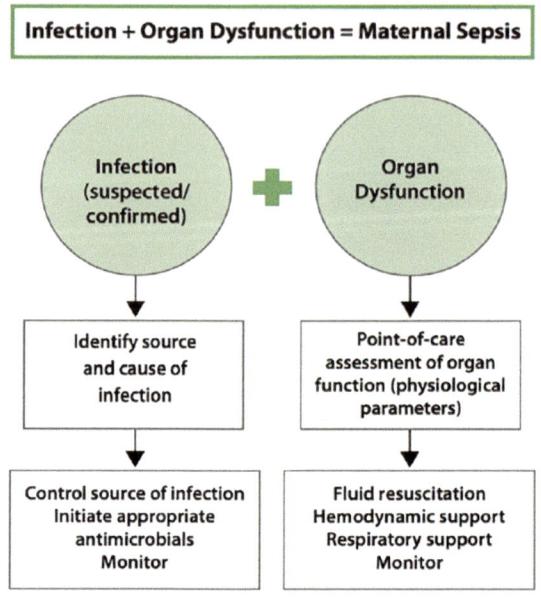

Table 8.1 New WHO definition of maternal sepsis

Definition of maternal sepsis—New WHO 2016 definition
Maternal sepsis is a life-threatening condition defined as organ dysfunction resulting from infection during pregnancy, childbirth, post-abortion, or the postpartum period

Reproduced from: WHO 2016 [2] Copyright 2024

Screening for maternal sepsis can also be done with the help of a tool called the obstetrical modified qSOFA (sequential [sepsis-related] organ failure assessment) score, or the **omqSOFA**. The omqSOFA requires only clinical parameters. Its evaluation can be performed quickly without waiting for laboratory results. An **omqSOFA ≥2** is a predictor of in-hospital mortality, and this woman should be seen as critically ill and managed accordingly (Table 8.2).

Call for help as soon as you suspect maternal sepsis, as the time elapsed until therapy is critical for survival!

The AVPU (alert, voice, pain, unresponsive) scale can be used to assess level of consciousness (Table 8.3).

You should quickly evaluate the possible source of infection (Table 8.4):

- **Infection of the uterus**:
  - Pregnant: Is the foetus tachycardic (>160 beats/min [bpm])? Did the woman have prolonged rupture of membranes and/or an intrauterine invasive procedure?
  - After birth: Does the woman have abdominal pain, distended abdomen, foul-smelling vaginal discharge, vaginal bleeding?

Fig. 8.2 Maternal sepsis: signs and symptoms. (Reproduced from: WHO 2017 maternal sepsis definition and management [3], Copyright 2024)

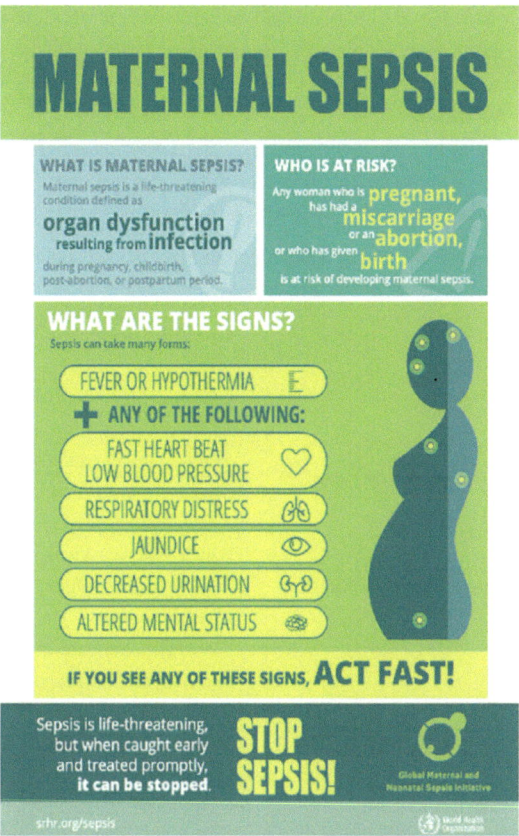

Table 8.2 Obstetrical modified qSOFA score [4]

Parameter	Score	
	0	1
Systolic blood pressure	≥90 mmHg	<90 mmHg
Respiratory rate	Less than 25 breaths/min	25 breaths/min or more
Altered mentation	Alert	Not alert

Copyright 2024 John Wiley and Sons
min minute, *mmHg* millimetres of mercury, *qSOFA* quick Sequential (sepsis-related) Organ Failure Assessment score

- **Wound infection**: Does the perineal wound or caesarean section scar look reddened, swollen, warm, and/or is it painful?
- **Urinary infection**: Does the woman have painful or burning micturition and/or back pain?
- **Mastitis puerperalis/breast abscess**: Does the breast show signs of infection (reddened, swollen, warm, painful)?

Table 8.3 AVPU scale for evaluation of level of consciousness [5]

Evaluation of level of consciousness: AVPU scale	
A—Alert	Alert and conscious
V—Voice	Responds to voice
P—Pain	Responds to pain
U—Unresponsive	No response to voice or pain

Table 8.4 Pathogens involved in maternal sepsis [4]

Infection	Pathogens
Bacterial—common	Group A-beta-haemolytic Streptococcus (GAS) pyogenes
	Escherichia coli
	Group B Streptococcus
	Klebsiella pneumoniae
	Staphylococcus aureus
	Streptococcus pneumonia
	Proteus mirabilus
	Anaerobic organisms
Bacterial—less common	*Haemophilus influenza*
	Listeria monocytogenes
	Clostridium species
	Mycobacterium tuberculosis
Viral	Influenza
	Varicella zoster virus
	Herpes simplex virus
	Cytomegalovirus

Copyright 2024 John Wiley and Sons

- **Respiratory infection/pneumonia**: Does the woman cough, have a severe sore throat, or dyspnoea?
- **Meningitis**: Does the woman have a severe headache and back pain or other neurological symptoms?
- Any other symptoms indicative of infection? At the same time, you should evaluate the woman for signs of gravity ('red flags'; Fig. 7.5). Therefore, you need to measure blood pressure, pulse, respiratory rate, and, if available, blood oxygen saturation. Ask the woman or if unconscious an accompanying person if the woman was able to pass urine in the last 18 h.

If one or more of the following **red flags** are present

- Responds only to voice or pain/is unresponsive
- Systolic blood pressure ≤90 mmHg
- Heart rate >130 bpm
- Respiratory rate ≥25 breaths/min
- Needs oxygen to keep oxygen saturation ≥92%
- Non-blanching rash, mottled/ashen/cyanotic skin

- Has not passed urine in last 18 h
- Urine output less than 0.5 mL/kg/h

then immediately start the therapeutic pathway '**Sepsis Six**' (Fig. 7.6).

8.1.1.2 Sepsis Management

The objective is to achieve the actions listed in the '**Sepsis Six**' pathway within **1 h** after first suspicion of sepsis. Call for help, medical doctor and/or anaesthetist if available!

- Give oxygen.
- Take blood cultures or other swabs (urine, vaginal, throat, if appropriate lumbar puncture, etc.) to confirm source of infection—think ahead about infection source control and timing of birth!
- Perform blood tests: full blood count, urea and electrolytes, liver function tests, and clotting (and lactate if available).
- Give IV antibiotics according to local protocol. **Consider allergies before administration!**
- Give IV fluids (normal saline) up to 30 mL/kg (about 2 L).
- Measure urine output.
- Monitor respiratory rate, blood pressure, pulse, and blood oxygen saturation.
- Monitor foetal heart rate (intermittent auscultation).

8.1.1.3 Antibiotics

Administration of IV broad-spectrum antibiotics is recommended **within 1 h of suspicion of severe sepsis**, with or without septic shock. Mortality increases by 7.6% with each hour delay in appropriate antibiotic administration in the general population. Examples of antibiotic treatments can be found in [6].

Depending on the source of infection, more actions may be needed after the first assessment and initial stabilization of the woman. Infection source control may require the following interventions:

- If chorioamnionitis is suspected: Plan to deliver the baby (induction of labour or caesarean section).
- If retained products or incomplete placenta is suspected: Curettage may be needed.
- If breast abscess or other wound abscess is suspected: Incision and/or drainage may be needed.
- If pneumonia is suspected: Consider chest X-ray.

A woman may also present earlier in the course of infection. In this case, she may present with less severe signs and symptoms but should still be thoroughly assessed and given prompt therapy. This will prevent infection from spreading

further and endangering the life of the mother and her baby. These **less severe signs and symptoms** are described as '**amber flags**' and are listed here and in Fig. 8.3:
   Amber flags for sepsis:

- Relatives concerned about the mother's mental status
- Acute deterioration in functional ability
- Respiratory rate 21–24 breaths/min *or* breathing hard
- Heart rate 100–130 bpm *or* new arrhythmia
- Systolic BP 91–100 mmHg
- Has not passed urine in last 12–18 h
- Temperature <36 °C
- Has had invasive procedure in the last 6 weeks (caesarean section, miscarriage, others)
- Prolonged rupture of membranes
- Bleeding/wound infection/vaginal discharge
- Non-reassuring foetal heart rate/foetal tachycardia >160 bpm

8.1.1.4   Follow-Up Care

The woman is very likely to need intensive monitoring of blood pressure, pulse, temperature, and urinary output to adapt fluid management and ensure timely administration of further doses of antibiotics. A woman with sepsis should stay at a place within the hospital where this monitoring can be guaranteed (obstetrics ward, intensive care unit if available).

8.1.1.5   Examination of the Newborn

If there is a suspicion of chorioamnionitis as a cause of sepsis, the newborn also has a high risk of infection and should be examined by a paediatrician very soon after birth. If the woman has not given birth yet, it may become necessary to expedite birth by induction of labour or caesarean section.

8.1.1.6   Preventing Infection and Sepsis

A detailed description of preventive actions for infection and sepsis is beyond this manual's scope. However, it is essential to remember that simple rules such as regular handwashing with water and soap or antiseptic solution and clean birth practices may have a significant effect on maternal and foetal infection prevention.

8.1.2   Algorithms

The recognition and management of maternal sepsis are described in Figs. 8.3 and 8.4, respectively.

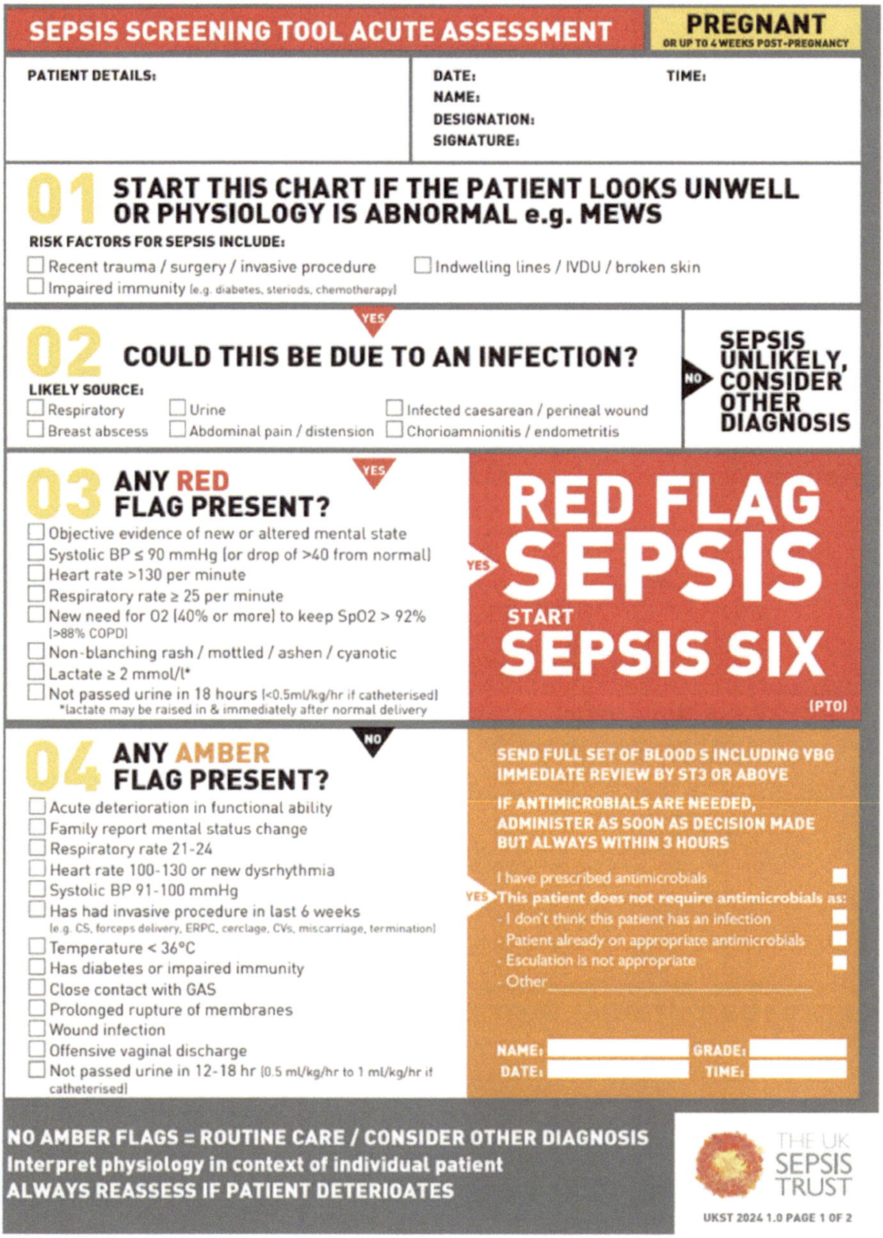

SEPSIS SCREENING TOOL ACUTE ASSESSMENT

PREGNANT
OR UP TO 4 WEEKS POST-PREGNANCY

PATIENT DETAILS:

DATE:
NAME:
DESIGNATION:
SIGNATURE:

TIME:

01 START THIS CHART IF THE PATIENT LOOKS UNWELL OR PHYSIOLOGY IS ABNORMAL e.g. MEWS

RISK FACTORS FOR SEPSIS INCLUDE:
- ☐ Recent trauma / surgery / invasive procedure
- ☐ Impaired immunity (e.g. diabetes, steriods, chemotherapy)
- ☐ Indwelling lines / IVDU / broken skin

YES

02 COULD THIS BE DUE TO AN INFECTION?

LIKELY SOURCE:
- ☐ Respiratory
- ☐ Breast abscess
- ☐ Urine
- ☐ Abdominal pain / distension
- ☐ Infected caesarean / perineal wound
- ☐ Chorioamnionitis / endometritis

NO → **SEPSIS UNLIKELY, CONSIDER OTHER DIAGNOSIS**

03 ANY RED FLAG PRESENT?
YES

- ☐ Objective evidence of new or altered mental state
- ☐ Systolic BP ≤ 90 mmHg (or drop of >40 from normal)
- ☐ Heart rate >130 per minute
- ☐ Respiratory rate ≥ 25 per minute
- ☐ New need for O2 (40% or more) to keep SpO2 > 92% (>88% COPD)
- ☐ Non-blanching rash / mottled / ashen / cyanotic
- ☐ Lactate ≥ 2 mmol/l*
- ☐ Not passed urine in 18 hours (<0.5ml/kg/hr if catheterised)
  *lactate may be raised in & immediately after normal delivery

YES → **RED FLAG SEPSIS START SEPSIS SIX** (PTO)

04 ANY AMBER FLAG PRESENT?
NO

- ☐ Acute deterioration in functional ability
- ☐ Family report mental status change
- ☐ Respiratory rate 21-24
- ☐ Heart rate 100-130 or new dysrhythmia
- ☐ Systolic BP 91-100 mmHg
- ☐ Has had invasive procedure in last 6 weeks
  (e.g. CS, forceps delivery, ERPC, cerclage, CVs, miscarriage, termination)
- ☐ Temperature < 36°C
- ☐ Has diabetes or impaired immunity
- ☐ Close contact with GAS
- ☐ Prolonged rupture of membranes
- ☐ Wound infection
- ☐ Offensive vaginal discharge
- ☐ Not passed urine in 12-18 hr (0.5 ml/kg/hr to 1 ml/kg/hr if catheterised)

SEND FULL SET OF BLOOD S INCLUDING VBG IMMEDIATE REVIEW BY ST3 OR ABOVE

IF ANTIMICROBIALS ARE NEEDED, ADMINISTER AS SOON AS DECISION MADE BUT ALWAYS WITHIN 3 HOURS

YES →
- I have prescribed antimicrobials ☐
- This patient does not require antimicrobials as: ☐
  - I don't think this patient has an infection ☐
  - Patient already on appropriate antimicrobials ☐
  - Esculation is not appropriate ☐
  - Other _____

NAME: GRADE:
DATE: TIME:

NO AMBER FLAGS = ROUTINE CARE / CONSIDER OTHER DIAGNOSIS
Interpret physiology in context of individual patient
ALWAYS REASSESS IF PATIENT DETERIOATES

THE UK
SEPSIS TRUST

UKST 2024 1.0 PAGE 1 OF 2

Fig. 8.3 Signs of gravity in maternal sepsis: red flags [7]. This document will not be updated in line with the updates of UK trust

SEPSIS SCREENING TOOL - THE SEPSIS SIX

PREGNANT
OR UP TO 4 WEEKS POST-PREGNANCY

PATIENT DETAILS:

DATE:
NAME:
DESIGNATION:
SIGNATURE:

TIME:

COMPLETE ALL ACTIONS WITHIN ONE HOUR

01   ENSURE ST3+ ATTENDS, CALL CONSULTANT
NOT ALL PATIENTS WITH RED FLAGS WILL NEED THE 'SEPSIS 6' URGENTLY.
A SENIOR DECISION MAKER MAY SEEK ALTERNATIVE DIAGNOSES/ DE-ESCALATE CARE.
NAME: GRADE:

TIME

02   OXYGEN IF REQUIRED
START IF O2 SATURATIONS LESS THAN 92% - AIM FOR O2 SATURATIONS OF 94-98%
IF AT RISK OF HYPERCARBIA AIM FOR SATURATIONS OF 88-92%

TIME

03   SEND BLOODS INCLUDING CULTURES
BLOOD CULTURES, VBG, BLOOD GLUCOSE, LACTATE, FBC, U&Es, LFTs, CRP AND CLOTTING
LUMBAR PUNCTURE IF INDICATED, CONSIDER RAPID PATHOGEN ID

TIME

04   GIVE IV ANTIBIOTICS, CONSIDER DELIVERY
MAX. DOSE BROAD SPECTRUM THERAPY (CONSIDER ESCALATION IF ALREADY ON ANTIBIOTICS)
CONSIDER: LOCAL POLICY / ALLERGY STATUS / ANTIVIRALS
EVALUATE NEED FOR IMAGING/ SPECIALIST REVIEW TO HELP IDENTIFY SOURCEIF SOURCE
AMENABLE TO DRAINAGE ENSURE ACHIEVED ASAP BUT ALWAYS WITHIN 12H

TIME

05   GIVE IV FLUIDS
IF LACTATE > 2mmol/L OR SBP < 90 mmHg GIVE 500mL over 15 min AND CALL
ITU REPEAT IF NO IMPROVEMENT.

TIME

06   MONITOR
USE EARLY WARNING SCORE e.g. MEWS. MEASURE URINARY OUTPUT: THIS MAY REQUIRE A URINARY
CATHETER. REPEAT LACTATE HOURLY IF INITIAL LACTATE HIGH OR CLINICAL CONDITION CHANGES

TIME

RED FLAGS AFTER ONE HOUR - ESCALATE TO CONSULTANT NOW
Monitor at least every 30 mins using early warning score e.g. MEWS

RECORD ADDITIONAL NOTES HERE:
e.g. allergy status, arrival of specialist teams, de-escalation of care, delayed antimicrobial decision making,
variance

The controlled copy of this document is maintained by The UK Sepsis Trust. Any copies of this document held outside of that area, in whatever format (e.g.
paper, email attachment) are considered to have passed out of control and should be checked for currency and validity. The UK Sepsis Trust registered charity
number (England & Wales) 1158843 (Scotland) SC050277. Company registration number 3644039. Sepsis Enterprises Ltd. company number 9583335. VAT reg
number 293113340E.

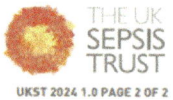

THE UK
SEPSIS
TRUST
UKST 2024 1.0 PAGE 2 OF 2

Fig. 8.4 Management of maternal sepsis: sepsis six pathway [7]. This document will not be
updated in line with the updates of UK trust

8.1.3   Conclusion

Be aware of the possibility of a woman having sepsis in pregnancy and up to six weeks after. The key points to a successful management are to recognise sepsis and act fast to treat it. Remember that these two key points may be challenging to achieve, as signs and symptoms of sepsis may be very unspecific.

References

1. WHO. WHO statement on maternal sepsis. WHO; 2017.
2. World Health Organization. WHO recommendations for prevention and treatment of maternal peripartum infections. WHO; 2015.
3. Global Maternal and Neonatal Sepsis Initiative. GLOSS the global maternal sepsis study. WHO; 2020.
4. Bowyer L, Robinson HL, Barrett H, Crozier TM, Giles M, Idel I, et al. SOMANZ guidelines for the investigation and management sepsis in pregnancy. Aust N Z J Obstet Gynaecol. 2017;57(5):540–51.
5. McNarry AF, Goldhill DR. Simple bedside assessment of level of consciousness: comparison of two simple assessment scales with the Glasgow Coma scale. Anaesthesia. 2004;59(1):34–7.
6. Shields A, de Assis V, Halscott T. Top 10 pearls for the recognition, evaluation, and management of maternal sepsis. Obstet Gynecol. 2021;138(2):289–304.
7. The UK Sepsis Trust. 2020.

Open Access   This chapter is licensed under the terms of the Creative Commons Attribution 4.0 International License (http://creativecommons.org/licenses/by/4.0/), which permits use, sharing, adaptation, distribution and reproduction in any medium or format, as long as you give appropriate credit to the original author(s) and the source, provide a link to the Creative Commons license and indicate if changes were made.

The images or other third party material in this chapter are included in the chapter's Creative Commons license, unless indicated otherwise in a credit line to the material. If material is not included in the chapter's Creative Commons license and your intended use is not permitted by statutory regulation or exceeds the permitted use, you will need to obtain permission directly from the copyright holder.

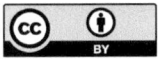

Chapter 9
Shoulder Dystocia

9.1 Introduction: Background and Evidence

9.1.1 Definition

Shoulder dystocia is defined as a vaginal cephalic delivery that requires additional obstetric manoeuvres to deliver the foetus after the head has been delivered and gentle traction has failed. Usually, the anterior shoulder impacts behind the maternal symphysis. Less commonly, the posterior shoulder impacts on the sacral promontory [5]. Figures 9.1 and 9.2 depict the mechanisms of shoulder dystocia.

Shoulder dystocia is an unpredictable obstetric emergency with potentially dramatic consequences. Its incidence is estimated to be around 0.6–0.7% of vaginal deliveries. Even with proper management, shoulder dystocia can be associated with considerable maternal and neonatal morbidity and mortality. Nevertheless, it is estimated that maternal and neonatal injuries in almost half of the cases were caused by substandard care and could have been avoided. It is very important to identify risk factors before and during childbirth, although every health care provider involved in childbirth must be prepared for this eventuality and be able to apply the necessary measures at any time. Risk factors are listed in Table 9.1.

One way of picturing the situation is to imagine the trailer of a truck impacted under a bridge, while the driver continues to apply the throttle, which only makes the problem worse. Similarly, pulling on the foetal head while the shoulder is impacted behind the symphysis does not release the newborn. On the contrary, excessive traction causes dangerous distention of the nerves coming from the cervical spine (a group of nerves called the brachial plexus) to innervate the arm (Table 9.2; Fig. 9.3). The result is damage or even tearing of the brachial plexus and paralysis of the child's arm and hand in internal rotation and adduction (Fig. 9.4). Rarely, brachial plexus paresis occurs after caesarean delivery by the same mechanism. Plexus brachial injury occurs in about 2–16% of shoulder dystocia. Most instances resolve without sequelae, but about 10% have permanent disability of the

© The Author(s) 2025, corrected publication 2025
C. Monod et al., *Simulation Training for Obstetric Emergencies in Low-Resource Countries*, https://doi.org/10.1007/978-3-031-81931-5_9

Fig. 9.1 Mechanism of
shoulder dystocia: anterior
foetal right shoulder
impacted behind the
maternal symphysis

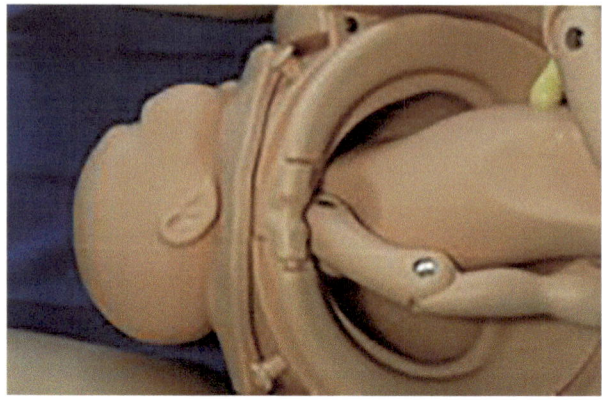

Fig. 9.2 Mechanism of
shoulder dystocia: anterior
foetal left shoulder
impacted behind the
maternal symphysis

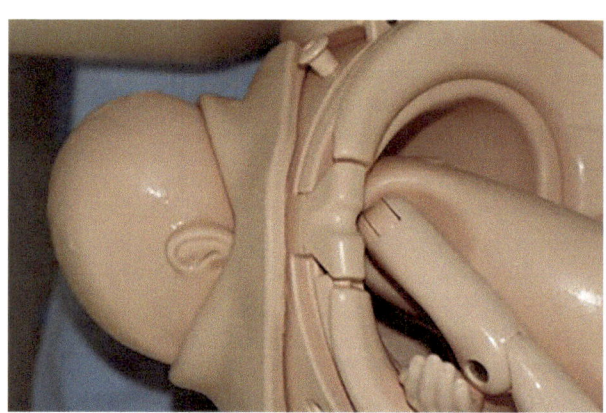

Table 9.1 Risk factors for shoulder dystocia [2] (Reproduced with permission of the Licensor through PLSclear)

Pre-labour	Intrapartum
Previous shoulder dystocia	Prolonged first stage
Macrosomia	Prolonged second stage
Gestational age	Labour augmentation
Maternal diabetes mellitus	Operative vaginal birth (forceps or vacuum)
Maternal obesity	

Table 9.2 Definition: brachial plexus nerves (adapted from [6])

Definition: brachial plexus nerves
Brachial plexus nerves are a bundle of nerves leading from the spinal cord to the shoulder and arm. This group of nerves controls the muscles of the shoulder, elbow, wrist, and hand, as well as the sensitivity in the arm

Fig. 9.3 Stretching of brachial plexus nerves in shoulder dystocia

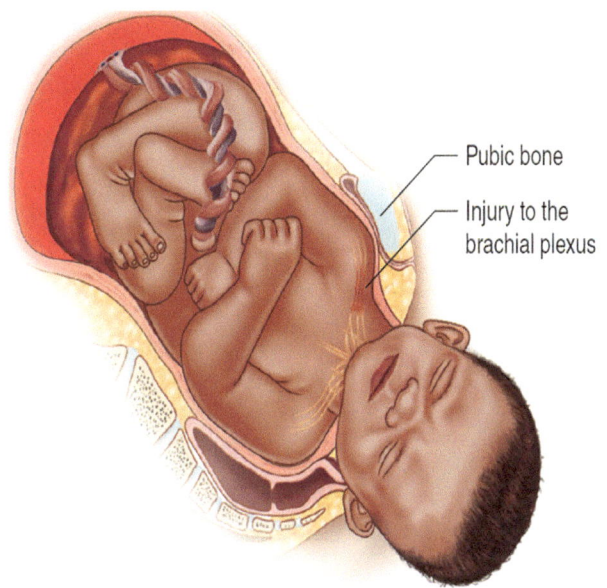

— Pubic bone

— Injury to the brachial plexus

arm and hand. Shoulder dystocia is associated with perinatal asphyxia and cerebral palsy. The risk of perinatal asphyxia increases with the time until resolution of shoulder dystocia and birth of the baby. Although it is not possible to determine precisely the time after which hypoxic complications occur, it appears that the rate of hypoxic ischaemic injury is low if the problem is resolved within 5 min. Therefore, the goal is to allow delivery of the child within 5 min of head birth. The hypoxic ischaemic encephalopathy is defined in Table 9.3. Maternal and other neonatal complications are listed in Table 9.4.

> **Timeline**
> To avoid ischaemic hypoxic consequences in the newborn, the aim is to resolve the shoulder dystocia and allow the birth of the baby within 5 min after the head.
>   **Deliver the baby within 5 min!**

Fig. 9.4 Arm position in
brachial plexus palsy

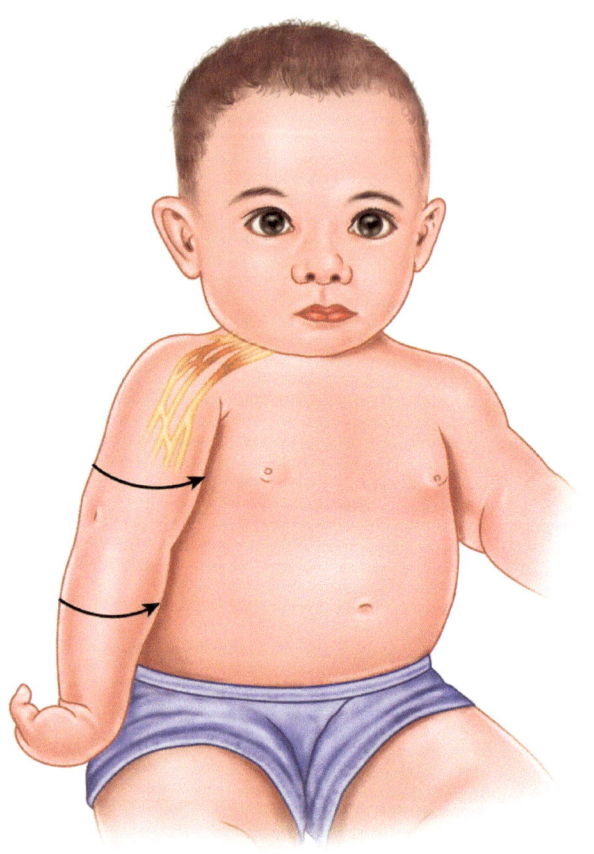

Table 9.3 Definition: hypoxic ischaemic encephalopathy (HIE) [1]

Definition: hypoxic ischaemic encephalopathy (HIE)
HIE is brain damage occurring when the brain does not receive enough oxygen or blood flow for a certain period. Hypoxic means not enough oxygen. Ischaemic means not enough blood flow. Children affected by HIE during the perinatal period, e.g. during birth, can present mild to severe neurological disability, such as epilepsy, cerebral palsy, or cognitive impairment

Table 9.4 Maternal and neonatal complications of shoulder dystocia [2, 5]

Maternal morbidity	Neonatal morbidity
Postpartum haemorrhage (11%)	Brachial plexus injury
Third- and fourth-degree perineal tears (3.8%)	Bone injury
Cervical tear	Hypoxic ischaemic injury (cerebral palsy)
Vaginal laceration	
Uterine rupture	
Bladder and urethral rupture	
Psychological birth trauma	

9.2 Management

9.2.1 Recognizing Shoulder Dystocia

The first step in the correct management of shoulder dystocia is recognising the problem.

Signs of shoulder dystocia are as follows:

- Difficulty with the birth of the face or chin
- Turtle-neck sign (incomplete expulsion of the foetal head, so that the foetal mandible and occiput remain depressing the maternal perineum. In the same way that a turtle retracts its head inside its shell) (Fig. 9.5)
- Failure of the restitution movement of the head
- Failure of the shoulder to descend

9.2.2 Routine Traction

Routine traction in line with the axis of the foetal spine can be applied for diagnosis, but **any other kind of traction MUST be avoided**. Downward or lateral traction distends the brachial plexus nerves and increases the risk of damage to them.

9.2.3 Call for Additional Help

Call for additional help as soon as you have identified the problem. Call the most experienced midwife available and, if possible, an obstetrician, paediatrician, and anaesthetist. Prepare for one health care professional to be available to take care of the newborn and to initiate resuscitation measures if necessary. As the team arrives,

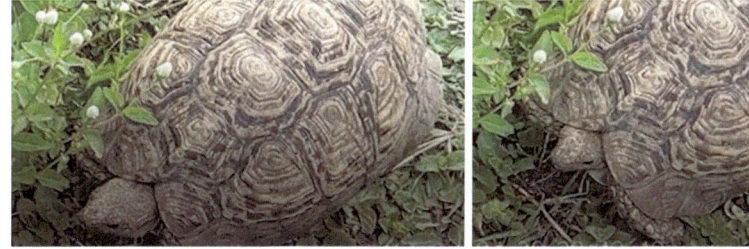

Fig. 9.5 Turtle-neck sign

state the problem loudly so that all team members know what is happening: 'We have a shoulder dystocia'.

9.2.4   Discourage Mother from Pushing and Stop Oxytocin

The mother should stop pushing, and you should stop oxytocin to avoid further impaction of the foetal shoulder behind the symphysis. In the same way, fundal pressure makes the problem worse and exposes the mother to the risk of uterine rupture.

9.2.5   Perform the McRoberts Manoeuvre and Apply Suprapubic Pressure

The McRoberts manoeuvre (Fig. 9.6) is a simple and effective method to relieve shoulder dystocia and should be used as the first manoeuvre. The success rate is as high as 90%! You need an assistant to perform it. It can be combined with suprapubic pressure to help the anterior shoulder rotate and slide under the symphysis.

9.2.5.1   How to Perform the McRoberts Manoeuvre

- Lay the woman flat; any pillows under her back should be removed.
- Each birth attendant holds one leg of the woman and first stretches the leg and then hyperflexes the thighs on her abdomen.
- Repeat the manoeuvre two to three times.
- Try to deliver the baby by applying routine axial traction on its head.

9.2.5.2   How to Perform Suprapubic Pressure

- Ideally from the side of the foetal back
- Just above the maternal symphysis
- In a downward and lateral direction
- Either in a continuous or with a 'rocking' movement

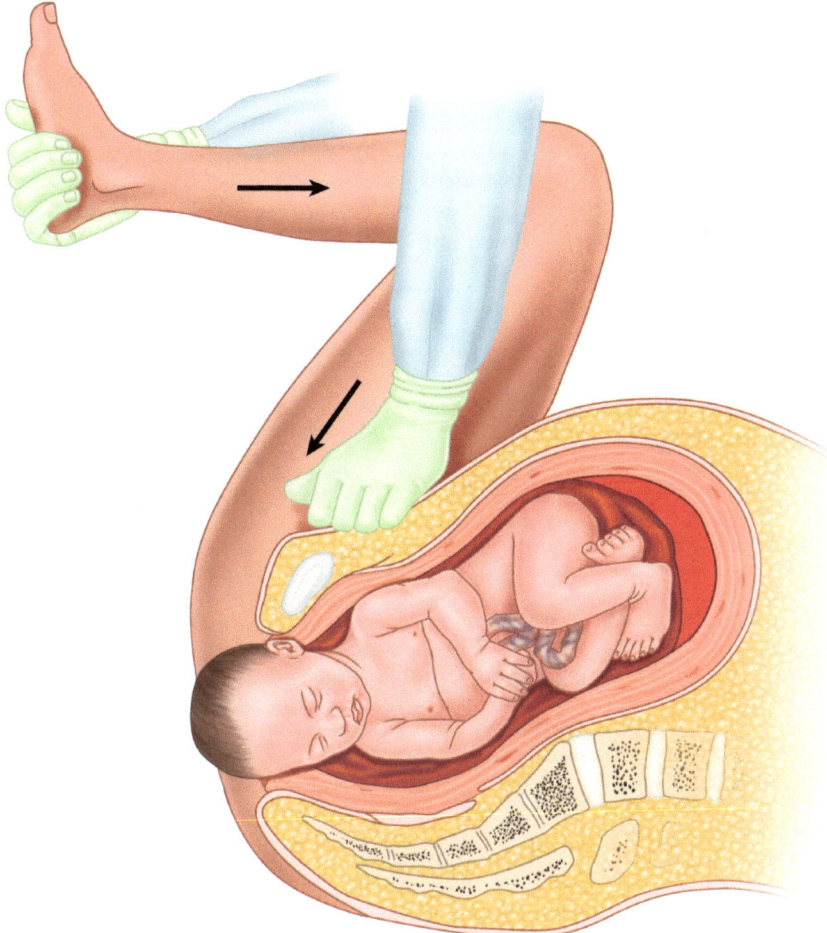

Fig. 9.6 McRoberts manoeuvre and suprapubic pressure

9.2.6 *When to Perform an Episiotomy*

An episiotomy should be considered to allow internal vaginal access for the whole hand of the birth attendant to perform manoeuvres. If access is easy without an episiotomy, it is not needed, but this should be documented in the woman's birth file. Shoulder dystocia is a **bony problem** that will not be resolved by an episiotomy.

9.2.7   What to Do Next If Simple Manoeuvres Fail? Internal Manoeuvres

9.2.7.1   Gaining Vaginal Access

Vaginal access should be gained **posteriorly.** The reason is that the sacral hollow is the most spacious part of the maternal pelvis. The access should also be achieved with the whole hand, folded as shown in Figs. 9.7 and 9.8. The woman should be moved to the edge of the bed.

Fig. 9.7 The whole hand

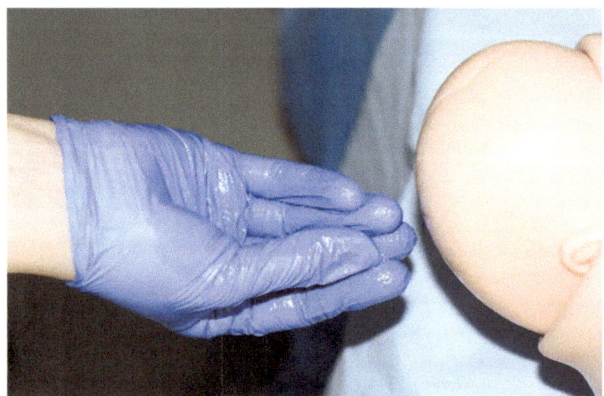

Fig. 9.8 Posterior vaginal access with the whole hand

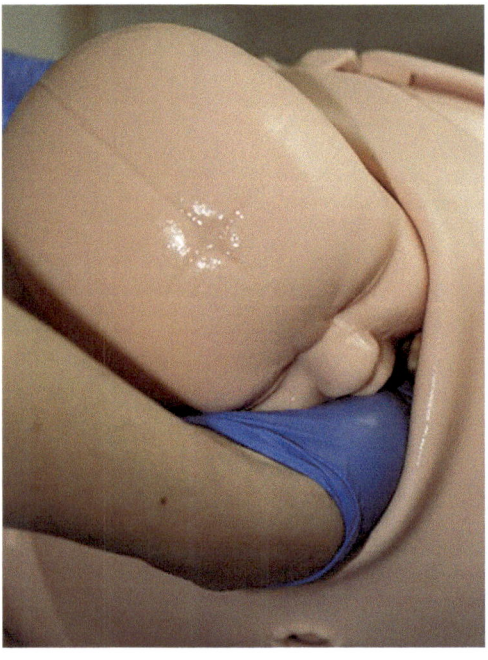

9.2.7.2 Rotation Manoeuvres

With the hand applying pressure on the posterior shoulder, ideally coming from the side of the foetal back, rotate the foetal body into an oblique diameter or best by a 180-degree rotation. Exerting pressure on the posterior aspect of the posterior foetal shoulder will reduce the diameter between the two shoulders, thus facilitating the release of the impacted shoulder. If this cannot be achieved, performing the rotation from the anterior aspect of the posterior foetal shoulder is possible (Figs. 9.9, 9.10, and 9.11).

Fig. 9.9 Internal rotation manoeuvres (1)

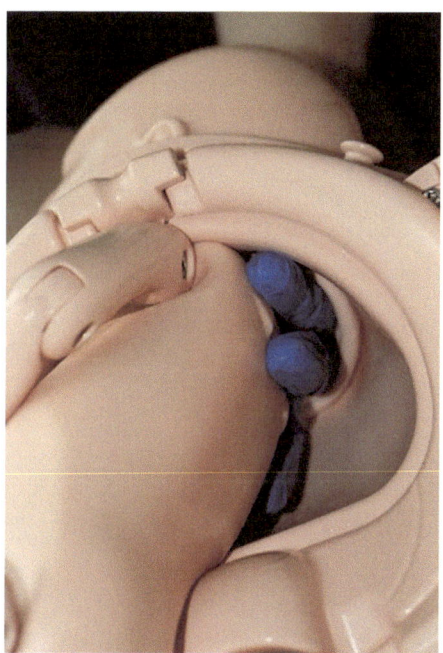

Fig. 9.10 Internal rotation
manoeuvres (2)

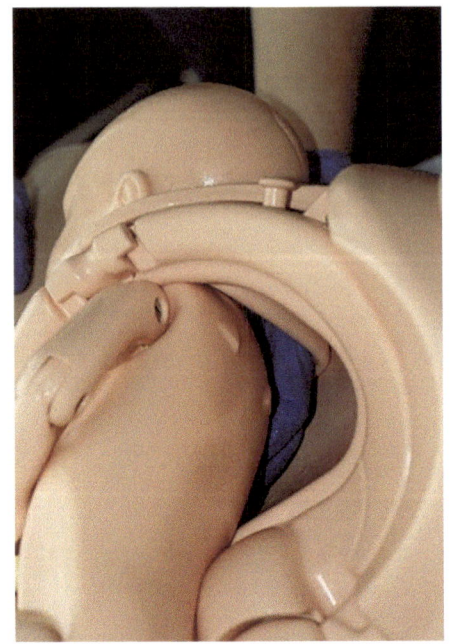

Fig. 9.11 Internal rotation
manoeuvres (3)

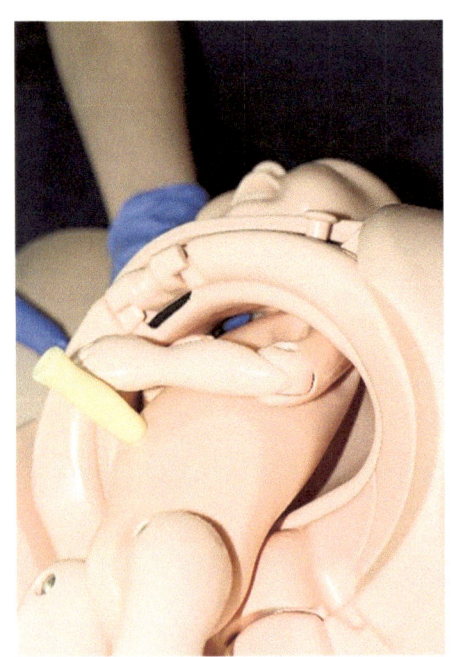

9.2.7.3   Delivery of the Posterior Arm

This manoeuvre reduces the diameter between the shoulders. The hand of the birth attendant grasps the foetal wrist and gently extracts the foetal arm out of the vagina by pulling in a straight line. Fractures of the humerus are seen in 2–12% of cases with this method, but it is unclear if this is due to the technique itself or to the refractory nature of the situation [3] (Fig. 9.12).

Fig. 9.12 Delivery of the posterior arm

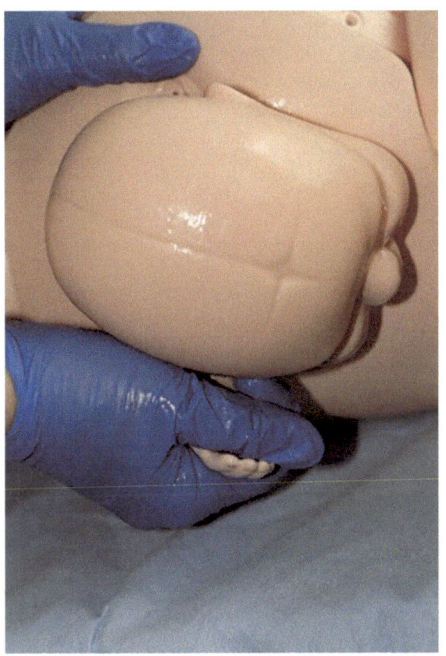

9.2.7.4   Posterior Axillary Traction

Although not included in many international guidelines, posterior axillary traction is well described in the literature and appears to have a satisfactory success rate and a low complication rate when performed correctly. In this manoeuvre, the birth attendant kneels in front of the birthing bed, introducing both hands' index finger into the posterior foetal axilla. A downwards pull is then applied in the direction of the mother's back to slide the anterior shoulder under the symphysis. It is imperative that the traction be exerted in this direction. Axial traction entails the risk of plexus brachial injury (Figs. 9.13 and 9.14).

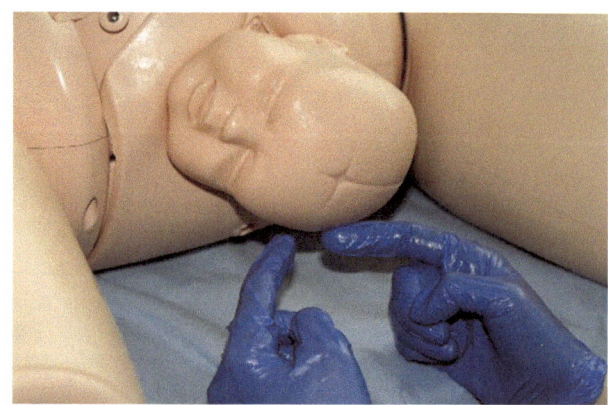

Fig. 9.13 Posterior axillary traction, position of the index fingers

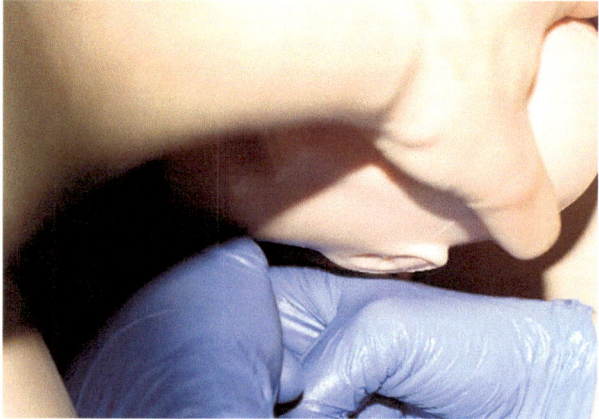

Fig. 9.14 Posterior axillary traction, elevation of the head

9.2.7.5 Delivering the Foetal Trunk

Once the manoeuvres have been successfully performed and the shoulder dystocia resolved, routine axial traction should be applied to deliver the foetal trunk. The mother can make gentle pushing efforts too.

9.2.8 What to Do Next If Simple Manoeuvres Fail? 'All-Fours' Position

Alternatively, a lean, well-mobile woman can position herself on all fours. This is a good alternative to internal manoeuvres, but which method is applied first depends on the situation and the experience of the birth attendant. Keep in mind that the goal is to achieve shoulder dystocia resolution within 5 min to avoid perinatal asphyxia.

9.2.9 Last-Resort Manoeuvres

Before moving on to the so-called last-resort manoeuvres, repeating the whole sequence from the beginning, ideally performed by another birth attendant, can still solve many cases. Last-resort measures have high perinatal and maternal morbidity and mortality. Fortunately, by being able to carry out the measures described above systematically, they are only necessary in exceptional cases.

It is unknown which is the most appropriate of the last-resort manoeuvres. We briefly describe the possibilities here.

9.2.9.1 Symphysiotomy

This measure means dividing the anterior fibres of the symphyseal ligament. Take care to protect the maternal urethra by placing a urinary catheter and displacing the urethra to the side with one hand. Palpate the symphysis to identify the symphyseal ligament and partly divide the fibres of the anterior symphyseal ligament. Note that maternal morbidity is high: urethral and bladder lesions, symphyseal separation, sacroiliac joint dislocation, or lateral femoral cutaneous neuropathy [3] (Fig. 9.15).

9.2.9.2 Vaginal Delivery After Abdominal Access

In this procedure, one birth attendant performs an emergency caesarean section and exerts pressure on the anterior shoulder to allow it to slip under the symphysis (Fig. 9.16). Another birth attendant delivers the baby vaginally. Vaginal internal manoeuvres can be performed concurrently with the abdominal efforts to deliver the baby.

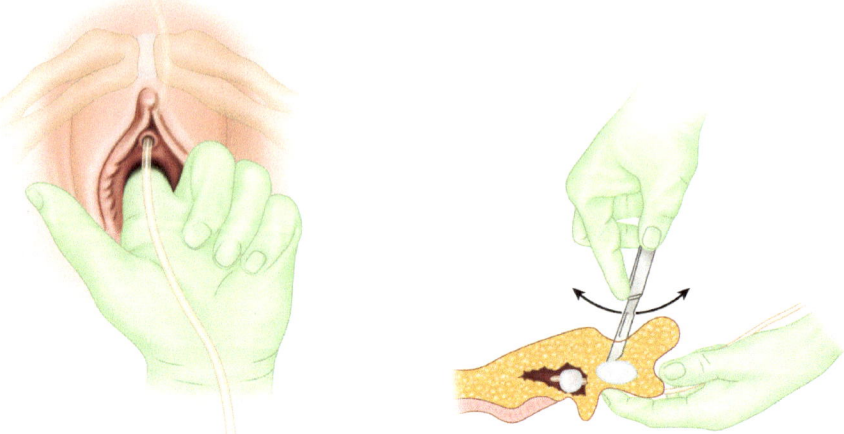

Fig. 9.15 Symphysiotomy [1]

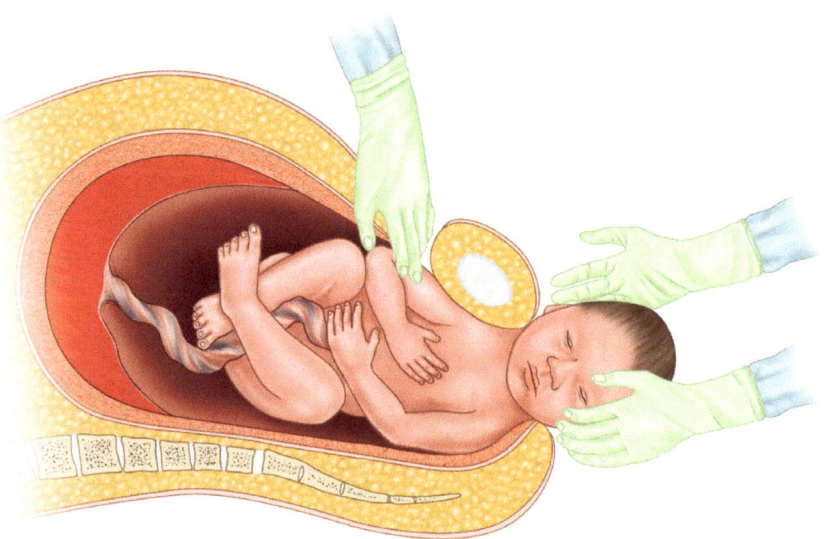

Fig. 9.16 Combined abdominal access and vaginal delivery in shoulder dystocia [4]

9.2.9.3   Vaginal Replacement of the Head (Zavanelli Manoeuvre)

In this manoeuvre, the child's head is pushed back into the mother's abdomen in the opposite way to the descent into the pelvis. The rate of maternal complications is not known, and severe foetal injuries are extremely frequent.

9.2.9.4   Cleidotomy

The birth attendant breaks the foetal collarbone with fingers or an instrument to reduce the diameter between the shoulders.

9.2.10   After Birth

9.2.10.1   Maternal Complications

There is a high risk of laceration of the birth canal, which can lead to significant blood loss and long-term maternal disability. Carefully check the vagina and perineum for high-degree perineal tears, cervical tears, or higher vaginal lacerations. Urethral injury and bladder and uterine rupture are all known complications. If necessary, do not hesitate to transfer the mother to the operating theatre to allow proper exposure and repair of the lesions. Seek help of a senior obstetrician if available and provide the mother with sufficient analgesia or anaesthesia. The risk of uterine atony and postpartum haemorrhage is also high so be prepared to handle this eventuality.

9.2.10.2   Neonatal Complications

A paediatrician should examine the newborn for bony and neurological injuries.

9.2.10.3   Communication with the Woman

It is essential to discuss the birth process with the woman. You should explain the course of events to her simply, in words she can understand. By doing so, you make an important contribution to the prevention of traumatic experiences of childbirth.

9.2.10.4   Documentation

Document carefully the sequence of manoeuvres you performed, why you did or did not perform an episiotomy, and if the right or the left shoulder was impacted, depending on the position of the foetus.

9.3   Algorithm

Figure 9.17 describes the management of shoulder dystocia.

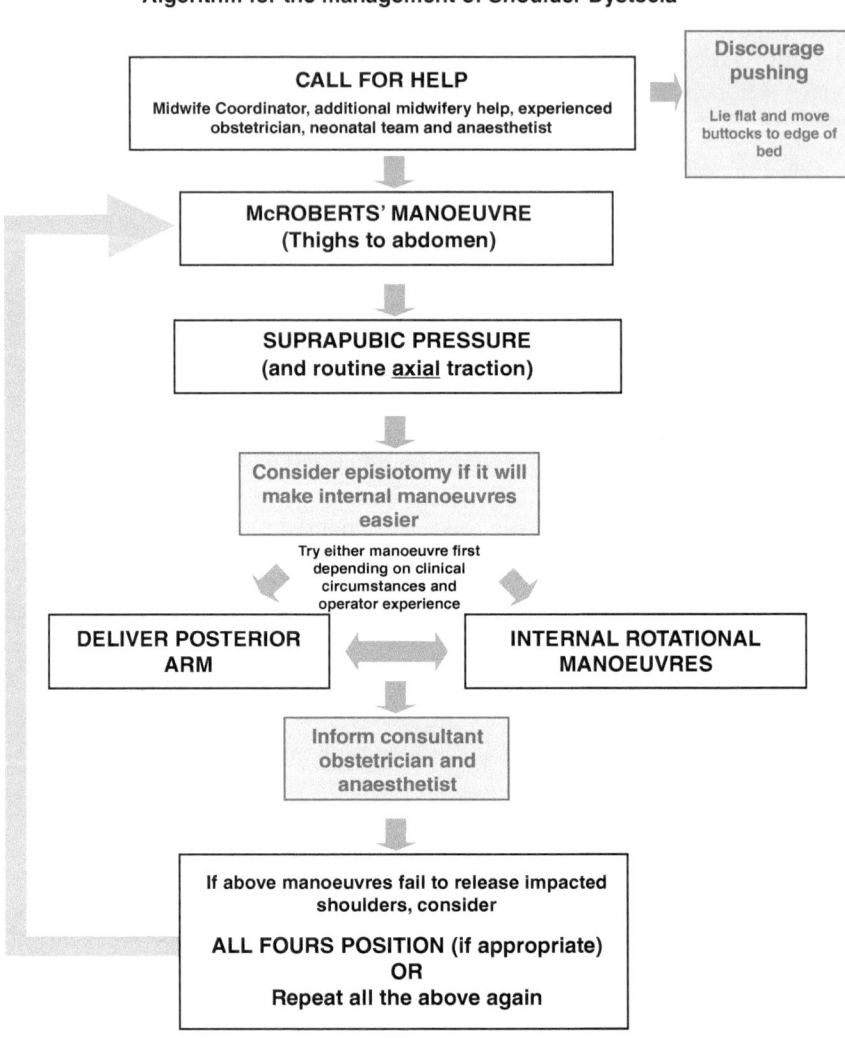

Fig. 9.17 Management of shoulder dystocia [5]. (Reproduced from: Royal College of Obstetricians and Gynaecologists. Shoulder Dystocia. Green-top Guideline No. 42 (Second edition). London: RCOG, March 2012, with the permission of the College. e52, with the permission of the College)

9.4   Conclusion

Shoulder dystocia is an unpredictable obstetric emergency, and every birth attendant should be prepared to cope with it at any time. Substandard care is responsible for the most long-lasting morbidity and mortality in both mother and child. In many cases, a skilled birth attendant can resolve the problem successfully by recognizing the problem early and performing the right manoeuvres systematically, thus minimizing maternal and neonatal morbidity and mortality.

References

1. California RotUo. Neonatal hypoxic ischemic encephalopathy.
2. Team TPE. PROMPT course manual, practical obstetric multi-professional training, 3rd ed. Cambridge University Press; 2017.
3. Gilstrop M, Hoffman MK. An update on the acute management of shoulder dystocia. Clin Obstet Gynecol. 2016;59(4):813–9.
4. Frontiers Ms. Medical guidelines.
5. Enekwe A, Rothmund R, Uhl B. Abdominal access for shoulder dystocia as a last resort—a case report. Geburtshilfe Frauenheilkd. 2012;72(7):634–8.
6. RCOG. Shoulder dystocia. Green-top guideline no. 42, 2nd ed. 2012.

Further Reading

Wikipedia. Brachial plexus. https://enwikipediaorg/wiki/Brachial_plexus.

Open Access This chapter is licensed under the terms of the Creative Commons Attribution 4.0 International License (http://creativecommons.org/licenses/by/4.0/), which permits use, sharing, adaptation, distribution and reproduction in any medium or format, as long as you give appropriate credit to the original author(s) and the source, provide a link to the Creative Commons license and indicate if changes were made.

The images or other third party material in this chapter are included in the chapter's Creative Commons license, unless indicated otherwise in a credit line to the material. If material is not included in the chapter's Creative Commons license and your intended use is not permitted by statutory regulation or exceeds the permitted use, you will need to obtain permission directly from the copyright holder.

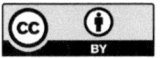

Chapter 10
Vacuum-assisted Birth

10.1 Introduction: Background and Evidence

Key Learning Points
- When performed safely, vacuum-assisted birth (VAB) may prevent unnecessary caesarean sections and complications in future pregnancies.
- Prerequisites for safe VAB are full cervical dilatation and ruptured membranes, accurate foetal station and position assessment, and a correct technique.
- It is important to place the cup correctly and to know how to identify the flexion point in VAB.

Operative vaginal birth (OVB) means assisting the vaginal birth of a baby with instruments. The first obstetric forceps were developed in the sixteenth century, and the first modern vacuum extractor in the mid-twentieth century. This chapter will describe how to use the Kiwi® Vacuum Delivery System, a plastic vacuum readily available to assist vaginal birth. Performing a VAB safely is a unique chance to improve neonatal outcomes and avoid unnecessary caesarean sections, thus preventing maternal complications in future pregnancies. However, VAB requires specific technical skills that may be challenging to acquire and maintain. Therefore, knowledge about indications, safety principles, and the instrument's practical use are prerequisites [3, 4].

Supplementary Information The online version contains supplementary material available at https://doi.org/10.1007/978-3-031-81931-5_10.

© The Author(s) 2025, corrected publication 2025
C. Monod et al., *Simulation Training for Obstetric Emergencies in Low-Resource Countries*, https://doi.org/10.1007/978-3-031-81931-5_10

10.1.1   Cervical Dilatation

The first prerequisites to perform a VAB are full cervical dilatation and ruptured membranes.

First condition for VAB is full cervical dilatation and ruptured membranes.

10.1.2   Classification

VAB is classified by the station and position of the foetal head. The station of the foetal head refers to the descent of the leading part of the skull within the birth canal, in relation to the maternal ischial spines. The position refers to the position of the foetal occiput in relation to the maternal pubic symphysis. The foetal station must be at least at the level of the ischial spines or below to fulfil criteria for safe VAB. Occipito-transverse and occipito-posterior positions are more challenging than occipito-anterior, as these foetal malpositions require rotation within the maternal pelvic cavity. VAB is subclassified into those with or without rotation. The second prerequisite to perform a safe VAB is to accurately assess the foetal station and position (Figs. 10.1, 10.2, 10.3, and 10.4).

Second condition for a safe VAB is a cephalic presentation and an accurate assessment of foetal station and position.

Foetal malposition (face and brow presentations) and breech presentation are all contraindications for VAB.

Fig. 10.1 Landmark of foetal skull

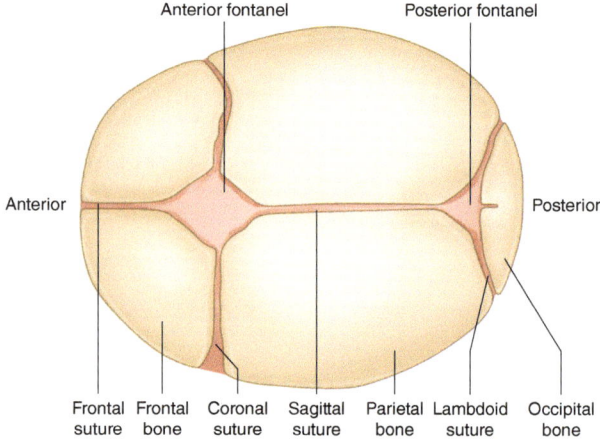

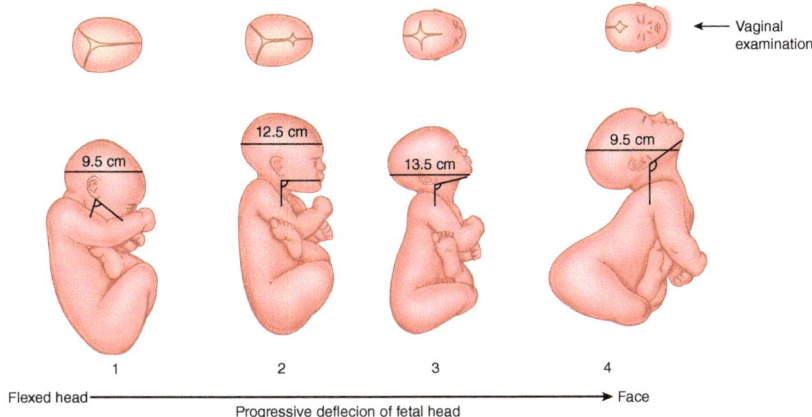

Fig. 10.2 Foetal head position: progressive deflexion

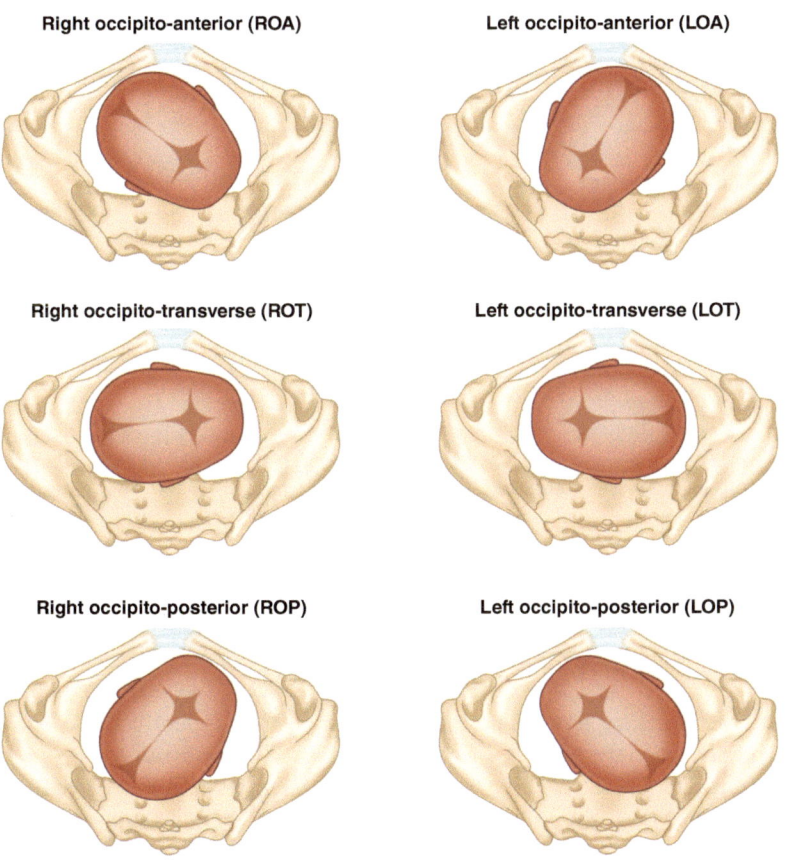

Fig. 10.3 Foetal head position (as in vaginal examination)

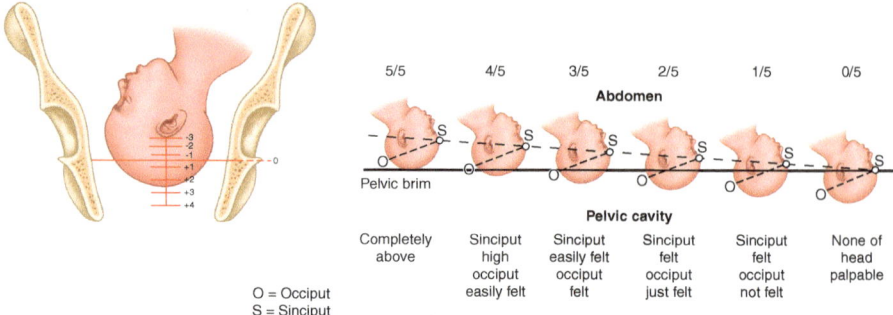

Fig. 10.4   Foetal head station in the vaginal and abdominal examination

Table 10.1 Classification of VAB [1] (Reproduced with permission of the Licensor through PLSclear)

Outlet	Fetal scalp visible without separating labia
	Fetal skull has reached the pelvic floor
	Sagittal suture is in the anterio-posterior diameter or right or left occiputo-anterior or -posterior position (rotation does not exceed 45°)
	Fetal head is at or on the perineum
Low	Leading point of the skull (not caput) is at station plus 2 cm or more and not on the pelvic floor
	Two subdivisions:
	• rotation of ≤45° from the occipito-anterior position
	• rotation of >45° including the occipito-posterior position
Mid	Fetal head is no more than one-fifth palpable abdominally
	Leading point of the skull is above station plus 2 cm but not above ischial spines
	Two subdivisions:
	• rotation of <45° from the occipito-anterior position
	• rotation of >45° including the occipito-posterior position
High	Not included in the classification as operative vaginal delivery is not recommended in this situation where the head is two-fifths or more palpable abdominally and the presenting part is above the level of the ischial spines

The classification of VAB is described in Table 10.1.

10.1.2.1   Indications

The decision-making process before performing a VAB is complex. VAB should be offered only when the benefits outweigh the risks. This evaluation may not be easy to perform. The first alternative to VAB is to let the mother push to give birth spontaneously. This may lead to foetal asphyxia or death if there is foetal compromise or even to maternal adverse outcome such as major PPH or deep perineal lacerations and fistulae if the expulsive phase last for hours. The second option is to perform a

Table 10.2 Indications and contraindications for VAB [1] (Reproduced with permission of the Licensor through PLSclear)

Type	Indication (relative)	Contraindication (relative)	Instrument-specific contraindication
Inadequate progress	Nulliparous: lack of continuing progress for 3 h[a] with regional anaesthesia or 2 h[a] without regional anaesthesia	Suspected cephalopelvic disproportion	
	Multiparous: lack of continuing progress for 2 h[a] with regional anaesthesia or 1 h[a] without regional anaesthesia		
Fetal	Presumed fetal compromise	Predisposition to fracture (e.g. osteogenesis imperfecta)	**Vacuum**: Gestation <34–36 weeks
		Malpresentation (brow, face mento-posterior)	Face presentation
			Fetal bleeding disorders
			Midcavity/rotational forceps: Fetal bleeding disorders
Maternal	Fatigue/exhaustion	Refusal to consent	
	Medical conditions that preclude maternal effort such as cardiac disease, hypertensive crisis, cerebrovascular disease		

[a] Total of active and passive second stage of labour

caesarean section at full dilatation, which also may be a complex intervention with higher risk of maternal and neonatal morbidity (haemorrhage, lacerations, extended hospital stay, uterine rupture, and placenta accreta in future pregnancies; neonatal admission to the neonatal care unit, neonatal trauma, etc.).

Table 10.2 describes current indications and contraindications for VAB. Several indications will often lead together to the decision to perform a VAB. For example, you may indicate a VAB in the situation of suspected foetal compromise in a woman who has been pushing for an hour. The decision to intervene depends on several factors, including the woman's preferences, and is always a balance between risks and benefits.

10.1.2.2 Complications of VAB

Complications are inevitable after any operative procedure, including after VAB, but they should be minimized by appropriate use and training. However, birth attendants should be aware that a failed evaluation of the clinical situation may lead to significant maternal and neonatal complications:

- Failure to diagnose a foetal malposition may lead to failed VAB.
- Ignoring signs of cephalopelvic disproportion or underestimating foetal weight in macrosomia may lead to failed VAB or shoulder dystocia.
- Second-stage caesarean section after failed VAB may be challenging due to the impaction of the foetal head in the maternal pelvis.
- Poorly conducted VABs is associated with high-degree perineal tears, vaginal wall and cervical lacerations, postpartum haemorrhage, and long-term pelvic floor sequelae. For the neonate, complications such as traumatic injuries, cerebral haemorrhage, or hypoxic-ischaemic encephalopathy may arise. These are, of course, all complications that may also arise by poorly conducted spontaneous vaginal birth or caesarean section. Consistent and systematic management is always essential to minimize them.

10.2 Management

Before performing a VAB, ensure that the prerequisites are fulfilled (Table 10.3).

10.2.1 Technique

Table 10.4 describes important landmarks for VAB, the flexion point and the midpoint of the foetal head.
The five steps of a VAB [2] (Figs. 10.7 and 10.8)

1. *Locate the flexion point and calculate the cup insertion distance*
Before inserting the vacuum cup

- Re-check the position of the occiput and flexion point.
- The cup insertion distance can be estimated with the help of the middle finger during the initial assessment.

2. *Hold and insert the cup*

- Gently retract the perineum with two fingers.
- The cup is inserted with one movement after a contraction.

3. *Manoeuvre the cup toward the flexion point*

- For low and outlet occipito-anterior positions, the flexion point will be in or near the introitus and little manoeuvring will be necessary.
- For mid- and low-pelvic occipito-posterior and occipito-transverse positions, the flexion point will be displaced away from the introitus toward the sacrum and manoeuvring of the cup will be necessary to achieve correct placement.
- Displacement of the flexion point in occipito-posterior and occipito-transverse positions is mainly in the antero-posterior direction of the birth canal and to a

Table 10.3 Prerequisites for VAB [1] (Reproduced with permission of the Licensor through PLSclear)

Prerequisites for operative vaginal delivery[a]	
Full abdominal and vaginal examination	• Head is no more than one-fifth palpable
	• Station at spines or below
	• Cervix is fully dilated and membranes ruptured
	• Diagnosis of the exact fetal head position (to ensure proper placement of instrument)
	• Assessment of caput and moulding (irreducible moulding may indicate cephalopelvic disproportion)
	• Pelvis is deemed adequate
Preparation of mother	• Clear explanation should be given and consent obtained
	• Appropriate anaesthesia
	• Maternal bladder should be emptied; indwelling catheter should be removed or balloon deflated
	• Aseptic technique
Preparation of staff	• Operator should have necessary knowledge, experience and skills necessary
	• Adequate facilities are available (appropriate equipment, bed, lighting)
	• Back-up plan in place in case of failure of OVB. When conducting midcavity births, theatre staff should be immediately available to allow a caesarean section to be performed without delay (<30 min), A senior obstetrician competent in performing midcavity OVBs should be present if a junior trainee is performing the birth
	• Anticipation of complications that may arise (e.g. shoulder dystocia, postpartum haemorrhage)
	• Personnel present that are trained in neonatal resuscitation

[a] Adapted from the Royal College of Obstetricians and Gynaecologists 2011

lesser extent lateral. For practical reasons, the vacuum cup should be manoeuvred in the axis of the maternal midline pelvis axis toward the flexion point.

• Ensure that maternal tissue has not been entrapped within the cup but take care not to dislodge the cup. It may not be possible to check for maternal tissue entrapment posteriorly in OP and OT positions, but the risk is very low as posterior vaginal tissue is very distended by the foetal head in this situation.

4. *Induce and maintain the vacuum*

• Build the vacuum until a pressure of 60–80 kPa is reached. If you are not sure if maternal tissue has been entrapped, pause after 20 kPa and check again before further building the vacuum.
• Start pulling gently in the next contraction in conjunction with maternal pushing efforts. Stronger traction should be delayed until the chignon (artificial caput succedaneum) has completely formed after about 1 min.

Table 10.4 Definitions: flexion point and midpoint of the foetal head [1] (Reproduced with permission of the Licensor through PLSclear)

Essentials: The flexion point and the midpoint of the foetal head
Flexion point
The flexion point is an imaginary point on the sagittal suture of the foetal scalp, 3 cm in front of (anterior to) the posterior fontanelle. It marks the exit point of the mentovertical diameter and is a critical landmark for VAB. When the centre of the vacuum cup has been placed over the flexion point and traction is applied, the foetal head diameter will be optimal for birth (e.g. the head will be moved in a flexed position). See Figs. 10.5 and 10.6
Midpoint
The midpoint of the foetal head is situated on the mentovertical diameter but within the cranium, approximately 6 cm from the vertex. The long axis of the foetal head pivots at the level of the midpoint as the head descends. Therefore, traction with a vacuum should not be applied upward until the midpoint has passed beneath the maternal symphysis. Since the midpoint is situated at same level than the widest diameter of the foetal head, the resistance to birth is greater at this level than at the level of the vacuum cup. The implication for practice is that when the vacuum cup has reached the vaginal introitus, the widest diameter of the foetal head is passing through the narrowest part of the birth canal, namely the pelvic floor and perineum. This phase of VAB is generally associated with more resistance levels than those encountered during the descent phase. See Fig. 9.17

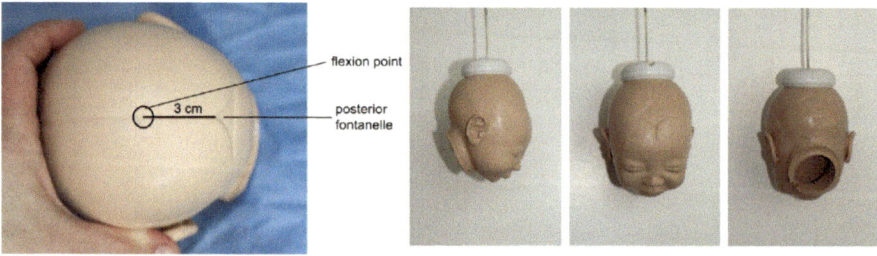

Fig. 10.5 Flexion point of the head and vacuum cup placement

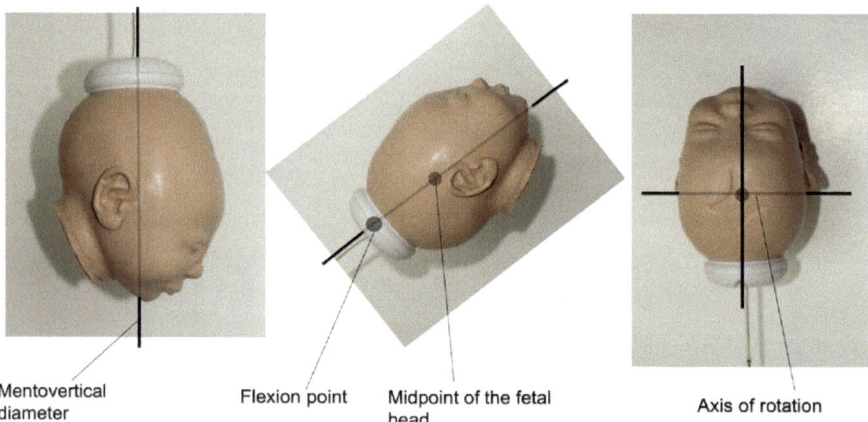

Mentovertical diameter   Flexion point   Midpoint of the fetal head   Axis of rotation

Fig. 10.6 Mentovertical diameter, flexion point and midpoint of the foetal head and cup placement

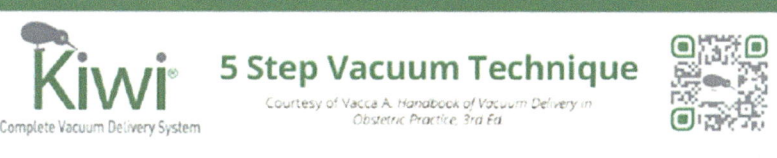

* Measure Length of Middle Finger

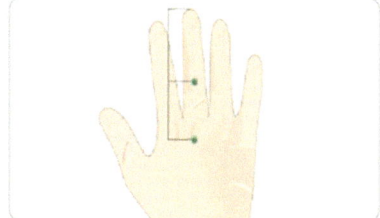

1 Locate Flexion Point & Calculate Distance

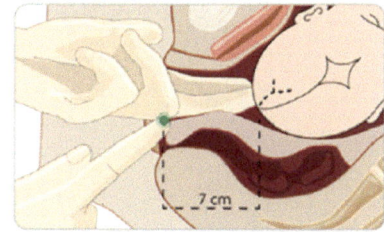

2 Hold & Insert Cup

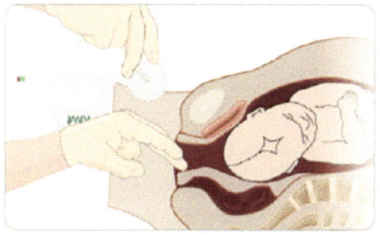

3 Move Cup Over Flexion Point

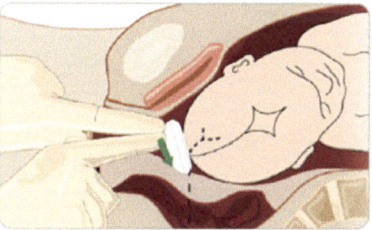

4 Create Vacuum & Exclude Maternal Tissue

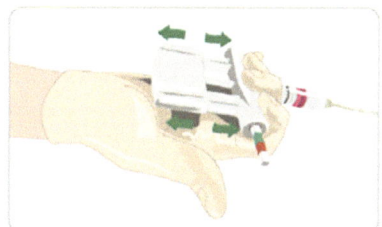

5 Initiate Traction

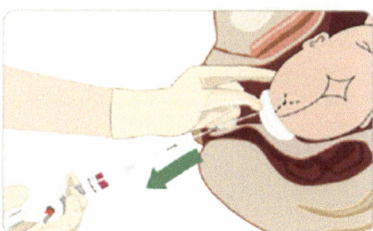

Fig. 10.7 Step vacuum technique permission from Laborie

5 Step Key Takeaways

1 Locate Flexion Point & Calculate Distance

Locate the flexion point. With opposite hand, note distance where finger meets introitus.
This is the distance you will insert the cup in step 3.

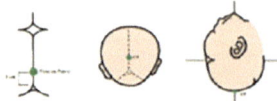

NOTE: The **flexion point** is located on the sagittal suture 3 cm forward of the posterior fontanelle.

2 Hold & Insert Cup

Hold cup with thumb on tube in groove, fingers on foam and insert into the vagina. After inserting, adjust cup so it lies flat against fetal head along midline.

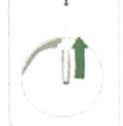

NOTE: Place 'groove' and stem of cup at **12 o'clock**. This allows one to visualize rotation as descent occurs.

3 Move Cup Over Flexion Point

Note 6 & 11 cm markings on stem tubing. Reference these markings to know how far to insert cup. Push cup **posteriorly along maternal midline** over flexion point. Insertion distance is the distance measured in Step 1.

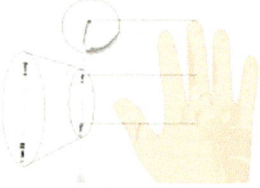

NOTE: The flexion point is along the midline.

Do not push cup laterally.

4 Create Vacuum & Exclude Maternal Tissue

Use palm pump to create vacuum. Once initial vacuum is created, feel around cup to exclude any maternal tissue. Then continue pumping vacuum to 600 mmHg.

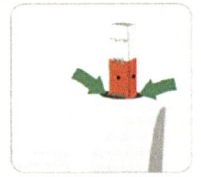

NOTE: Create vacuum to green section on gauge. If possible, 'bury' the green so it is no longer visible.

5 Initiate Traction

Initiate traction along axis of pelvis. Pull during contractions. Do **not move handle up and down or side to side while pulling.**

FINGER / THUMB TECHNIQUE
Use thumb and index finger of non-pulling hand to support the cup and the fetal head while pulling. This will help identify loss of vacuum before a pop-off occurs, while also providing feedback on descent.

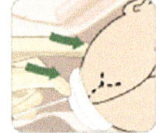

2 x 2 FINGERTIP GRIP
Ensure you have two fingers on the handle to each side of the stem. This helps with equal pulling while reducing likelihood of accidentally pressing the vacuum release button.

Correct   Incorrect

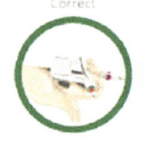   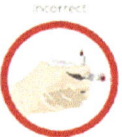

*Ruler

11 cm
10 cm
9 cm
8 cm
7 cm
6 cm
5 cm
4 cm
3 cm
2 cm
1 cm

Use ruler to measure distance from middle finger tip to ischial spinal point and metacarpal joint.

See Instructions for Use for full instructions, warnings, precautions & contraindications

Local Distributor:

clinicalinnovations.com
747 East 4170 South | Murray, Utah USA 84123
Phone +1 801 268 8200 | Fax +1 801 266 7373
Toll Free +1 888 268 6222

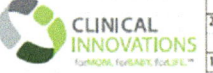
CLINICAL INNOVATIONS
forMOM, forBABY, forLIFE.™

Fig. 10.8   Five step key takeaways permission from Laborie

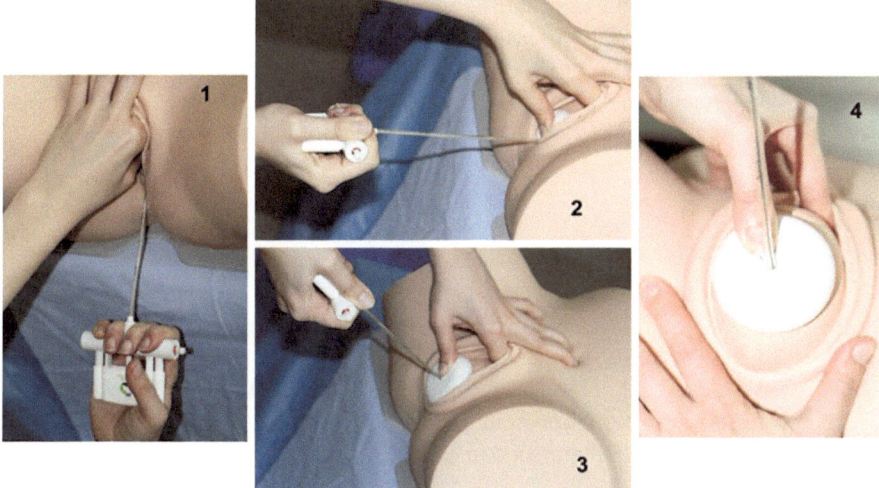

Fig. 10.9 Direction of traction in vaginal-assisted birth (VAB)

5. *Apply traction*

- The direction of traction should be first applied downwards, following the pelvic axis, always with maternal expulsive efforts (Fig. 10.9).
- For outlet VAB or when the head has descended to the outlet, the direction of traction will progressively change to an upwards direction.
- Cup attachment to the foetal scalp is more effective when the pulling direction is perpendicular to the cup.
- Traction is a two-handed action. The 'pulling hand' applies the traction, and the 'non-pulling hand' provides countertraction and prevents cup detachment.
- Traction should only be applied concomitantly with the contraction and maternal pushing effort. If uterus contractions are too weak, an oxytocin infusion should be started.
- Avoid rotating or side-to-side movement.

The 'fingertip' position of the pulling hand
The functions of the pulling hand are as follows:

- To direct the traction along the maternal pelvic axis to flex the foetal head, to achieve optimal presenting foetal head diameters for birth
- To provide additional but not excessive traction in addition to maternal pushing
- To limit the traction forces by pulling only with the fingertips and only during the contraction when the mother is pushing

The 'finger–thumb' position of the non-pulling hand

- The thumb of the non-pulling hand should be placed on the dome of the cup to provide some degree of counterpressure when needed during traction.

- The index finger of the non-pulling hand should rest on the foetal scalp in front of the cup and control progression (descent, flexion, autorotation). This finger–thumb position should be maintained until the head has crowned or delivered. Most cup detachments ('pop-offs') occur once the cup has reached the introitus. An assistant, not the operator, should provide perineal support.

10.2.2   Signs of Progress

Some progress should be visible with each pull. There should be a progression of the foetal head, not only of the scalp. The index finger of the non-pulling hand should feel the descent, flexion, and rotation. The traction tube of the vacuum will become progressively more apparent outside the introitus.

Two phases can be distinguished in VAB:

- The descent phase, from application of the cup until it is visible in the introitus
- The pelvic floor phase, until completion of birth

In many situations, a greater number of pulls are applied during the pelvic floor phase than in the descent phase. Traditionally, the 'three pulls rule' has applied to safe VAB. The rule states 'if there is not good progress after these three pulls, the case should be carefully reassessed'. However, a more modern practice may allow three pulls for the descent and three further pulls for the pelvic floor phase.

10.2.3   Cup Detachment or Pop-Off

Most cup detachments occur during the pelvic floor phase of VAB. The reason may be a cephalopelvic disproportion or a voluminous caput succedaneum. However, in most situations, an inadequate direction of traction is the cause. You may tolerate up to two cup pop-offs. After that, you should consider alternative measures, such as episiotomy if the birth appears imminent or caesarean section if not. Safety rules are described in Table 10.5.

Table 10.5 Safety rules: Know when to say 'STOP'! [2]

Know when to say 'STOP'!
If descent does not occur with each pull
If delivery is not achieved or imminent after three pulls
15–20 min total time limit
If the vacuum cup detaches (pop-off) more than 2 times

10.2.4   Episiotomy

Traditionally, an episiotomy was deemed mandatory for VAB. Nowadays, a restrictive use of episiotomy is recommended, and a routine episiotomy should not be performed. However, you may need some additional pulls to allow the perineum to stretch before completing the birth without an episiotomy. It is important to allow sufficient time for the perineum to stretch progressively.

10.2.5   After Birth

After the head is born, release the vacuum and complete the birth as usual. Inform the parents that the chignon on the newborn's head will disappear quickly. If the newborn is adapting well, give the newborn to the mother for bonding. Personnel for newborn resuscitation should be readily available in cases of VAB. Review maternal pelvic floor for tears after providing sufficient local anaesthesia. Explain the birth and intervention in simple words to the mother and answer her questions. The woman should urinate within 4 to maximal 6 hours after giving birth. If she is not able to do so, you should suspect urinary retention and catheterize the bladder. The risk of urinary retention also exists after a spontaneous vaginal birth but is increased after VAB.

10.3   Algorithm

The following Fig. 10.10 presents a flow chart for safe VAB. Note the use of a ABCDE mnemonic.

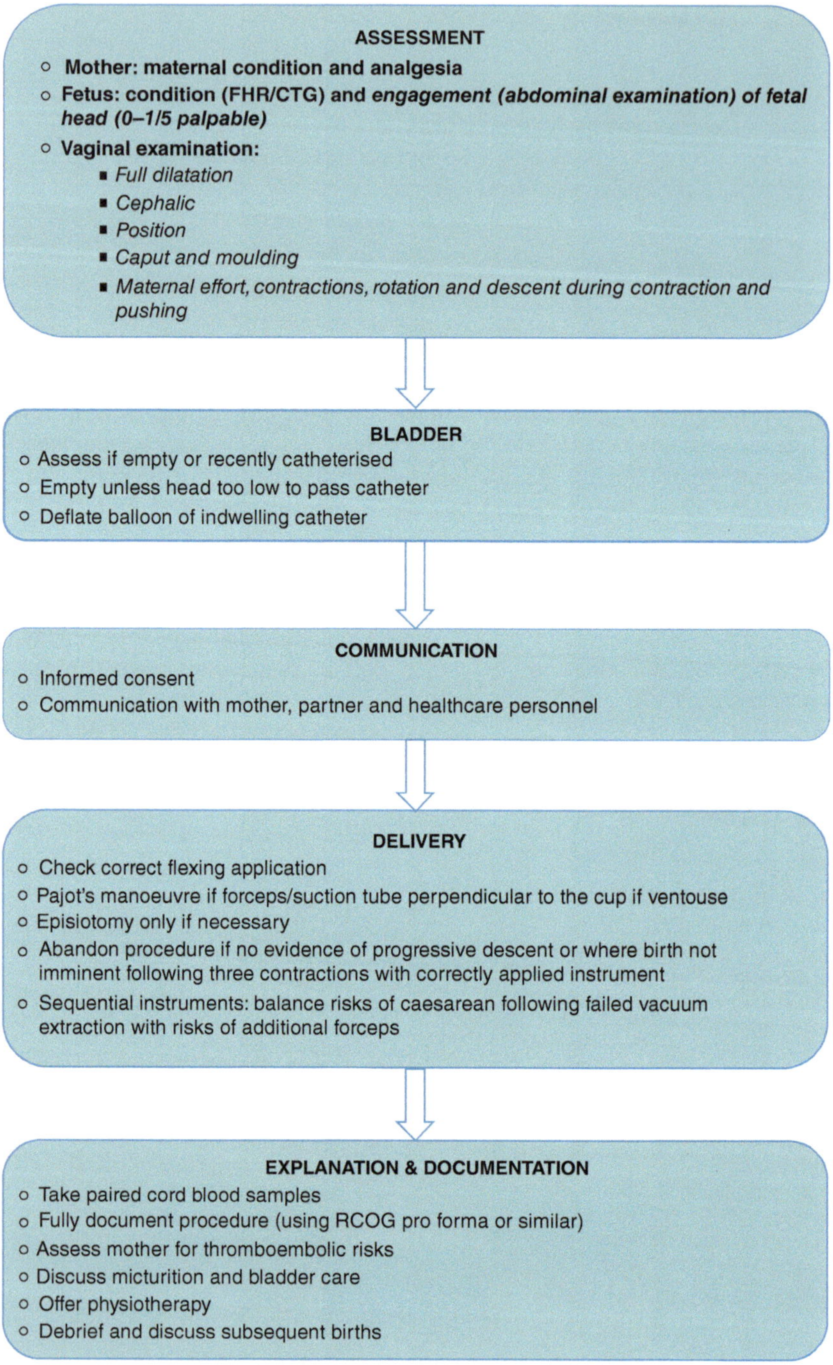

ASSESSMENT
- ○ **Mother: maternal condition and analgesia**
- ○ **Fetus: condition (FHR/CTG) and *engagement (abdominal examination) of fetal head (0–1/5 palpable)***
- ○ **Vaginal examination:**
  - ■ *Full dilatation*
  - ■ *Cephalic*
  - ■ *Position*
  - ■ *Caput and moulding*
  - ■ *Maternal effort, contractions, rotation and descent during contraction and pushing*

BLADDER
- ○ Assess if empty or recently catheterised
- ○ Empty unless head too low to pass catheter
- ○ Deflate balloon of indwelling catheter

COMMUNICATION
- ○ Informed consent
- ○ Communication with mother, partner and healthcare personnel

DELIVERY
- ○ Check correct flexing application
- ○ Pajot's manoeuvre if forceps/suction tube perpendicular to the cup if ventouse
- ○ Episiotomy only if necessary
- ○ Abandon procedure if no evidence of progressive descent or where birth not imminent following three contractions with correctly applied instrument
- ○ Sequential instruments: balance risks of caesarean following failed vacuum extraction with risks of additional forceps

EXPLANATION & DOCUMENTATION
- ○ Take paired cord blood samples
- ○ Fully document procedure (using RCOG pro forma or similar)
- ○ Assess mother for thromboembolic risks
- ○ Discuss micturition and bladder care
- ○ Offer physiotherapy
- ○ Debrief and discuss subsequent births

Fig. 10.10 ROBuST flow chart ABCDE: Vacuum-assisted birth algorithm [1] (reproduced with permission of The Licensor through PLSclear)

10.4 Conclusion

With a systematic approach and good technical skills, you may avoid unnecessary caesarean section by practicing safe VAB.

References

1. Attilakos GDT, Gale A, Siassakos D, Winter C. ROBuST: RCOG operative birth simulation training: course manual. Cambridge: Cambridge University Press; 2013.
2. Vacca A. Handbook of vacuum delivery in obstetrics. Vacca Academy; 2009.
3. Operative vaginal birth: ACOG practice bulletin, number 219. Obstet Gynecol. 2020;135(4):e149–ee59.
4. Murphy DJ, Strachan BK, Bahl R. Assisted vaginal birth: green-top guideline no. 26. BJOG. 2020;127(9):e70–e112.
5. Laborie. Vacuum assisted delivery proper cup placement. 2022. https://www.laboriecom/education/video-gallery/.

Open Access This chapter is licensed under the terms of the Creative Commons Attribution 4.0 International License (http://creativecommons.org/licenses/by/4.0/), which permits use, sharing, adaptation, distribution and reproduction in any medium or format, as long as you give appropriate credit to the original author(s) and the source, provide a link to the Creative Commons license and indicate if changes were made.

The images or other third party material in this chapter are included in the chapter's Creative Commons license, unless indicated otherwise in a credit line to the material. If material is not included in the chapter's Creative Commons license and your intended use is not permitted by statutory regulation or exceeds the permitted use, you will need to obtain permission directly from the copyright holder.

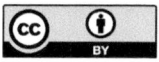

Chapter 11
Impacted Foetal Head at Caesarean Section

11.1 Introduction: Background and Evidence

In parallel with the overall increasing rate of caesarean sections, a rise in caesarean sections at full dilatation (CSFD) has been observed over the last few decades [8]. CSFDs are associated with a higher rate of maternal and neonatal complications because they can be technically challenging (Table 11.1) [13]. The risk of maternal death following emergency caesarean sections in the second stage is disproportionately high in low- and middle-income countries, and women in sub-Saharan countries [14].

Technical difficulties during CSFD arise from the following mechanisms:

- Foetal head is deeply impacted (Fig. 11.1) in the maternal pelvis, often in a deflected position like a ball in a pot.
- There is a vacuum between foetal and maternal tissues.
- The hand of the surgeon has no space between the foetal head and maternal symphysis.

These technical difficulties all lead to difficult foetal extraction and maternal and neonatal complications. Impacted foetal head may complicate as many as 1 in 10 emergency caesarean deliveries [2].

Supplementary Information The online version contains supplementary material available at https://doi.org/10.1007/978-3-031-81931-5_11.

© The Author(s) 2025, corrected publication 2025

C. Monod et al., *Simulation Training for Obstetric Emergencies in Low-Resource Countries*, https://doi.org/10.1007/978-3-031-81931-5_11

Table 11.1 Complications of CSFD and deeply impacted foetal head [1, 5, 6]

Maternal complications	Neonatal complications
Uterotomy tears (cervical, parametrium, corpus uteri)	Hypoxic ischaemic lesions
Ureter, bladder lesions	Bone injury
Vaginal lacerations	Intracranial bleeding
Postpartum haemorrhage	Peripheric nerve injury (brachial plexus palsy)
Infection (endomyometritis)	Spinal cord injury

Fig. 11.1 Deeply impacted foetal head in dorso-posterior-deflected-position

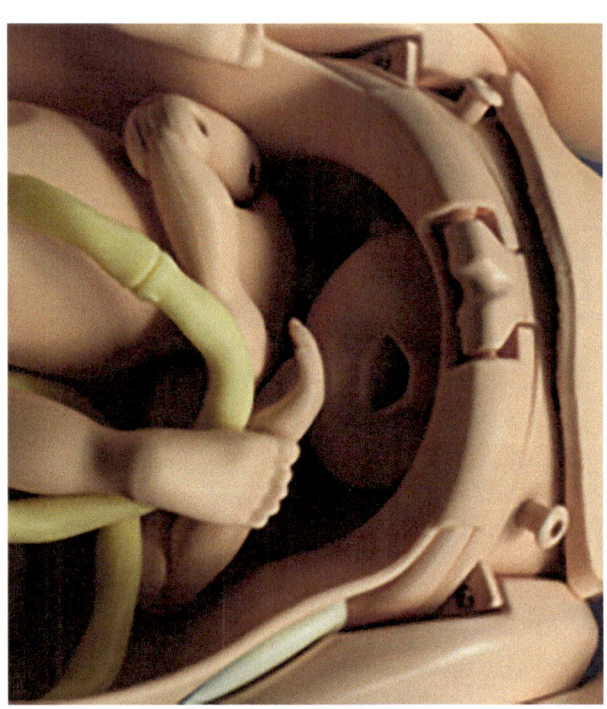

11.2   Management

This section describes how to manage CSFD to reduce maternal and neonatal complications [15].

11.2.1   Recognise Risk Factors [3]

It is essential to be aware of the risk factors for CSFD:

• Prolonged first and second stage of labour

- Long period of time between indication for caesarean section and the start of operation
- Foetal head deeply impacted in the maternal pelvis (interspinal)
- Deflected presentation (particularly in occipito-posterior presentation)
- Foetal macrosomia
- Maternal obesity (BMI > 30 kg/m^2)

11.2.2 Actions Before Proceeding to the Caesarean Section

- Stop oxytocin immediately after indication for caesarean section.
- Perform a vaginal examination again in the operating theatre just before proceeding to the procedure. If the foetal presentation is now low enough for operative vaginal delivery, inform the team and perform a VAB in the operating theatre.
- Be aware of foetal presentation; it will help with orientation in case of difficulties.
- Position the mother on the operating table with her legs slightly apart if vaginal access is needed.
- **Team Time Out**: Use the surgical safety check list [4] and inform the team of possible difficulties: difficult foetal extraction, risk of postpartum haemorrhage; if possible, inform the paediatric team.

11.2.3 Intraoperative Actions During CSFD

11.2.3.1 Initial Measures

- Position the operating table low enough or use a stepladder. It will allow a better angle to reach the foetal head and lower the risk of uterine tears towards the cervix and vagina (Fig. 10.3).
- In case of CSFD, perform a small bladder flap before uterotomy. It will help identify the structures in case of extension of the uterine incision towards the cervix.
- Place the uterotomy slightly higher than usual (about 2 cm) to avoid accidental extension of the uterine incision into the vagina. However, take care that the uterotomy still lies in the lower uterine segment.
- Insert the hand lateral to the foetal head if there is not enough space between the foetal head and symphysis (Figs. 11.2 and 11.3).

Gain lateral access to the foetal head if there is no space under the symphysis.

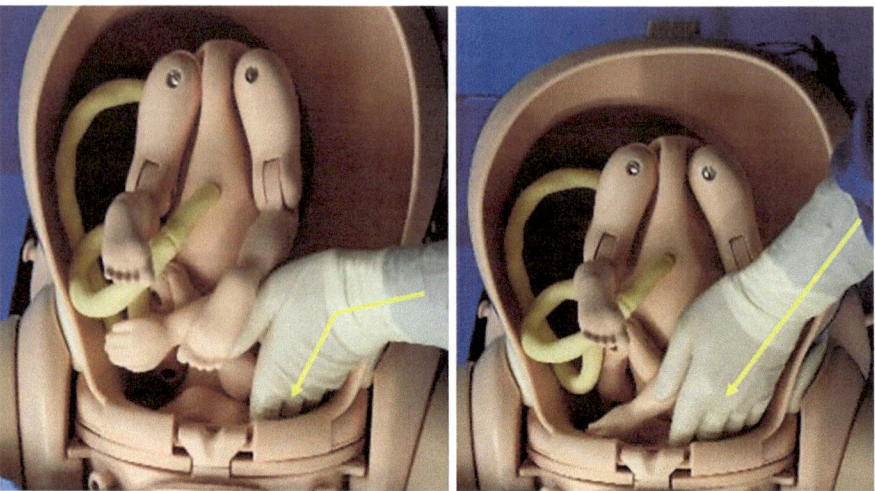

Fig. 11.2 Importance of positioning of the operating table at the right height

Fig. 11.3 Lateral access to
the foetal head

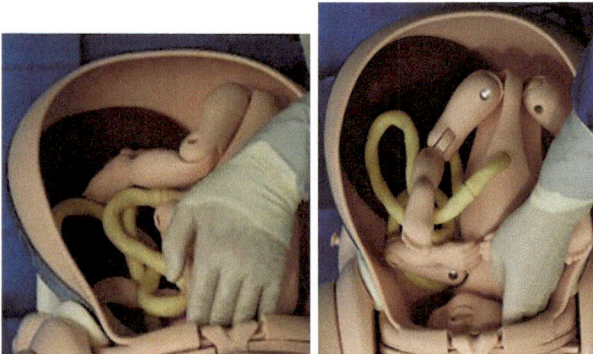

11.2.3.2   Technique to Deliver the Foetal Head

When delivering a deeply impacted foetal head during caesarean section, you must
respect the logic of birth mechanics to succeed. The movements the foetal head
must follow out of the pelvis are the opposite of those followed on the way down.
You can imagine an unscrewing movement to understand it better. It is essential to
release the vacuum, flex the foetal head, particularly when it is in an occiput posterior position before trying to push the head up and extract it out of the uterotomy
(Figs. 11.4 and 11.5).

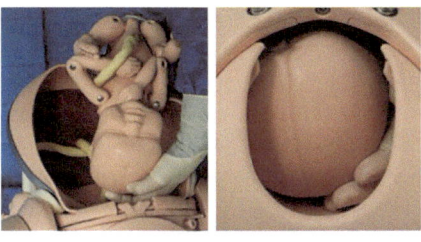

1. Relieving vacuum

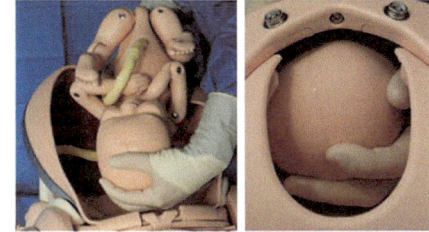

2. Flexion of fetal head

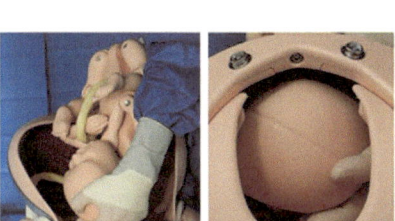

3. Rotation of fetal head in oblique
diameter

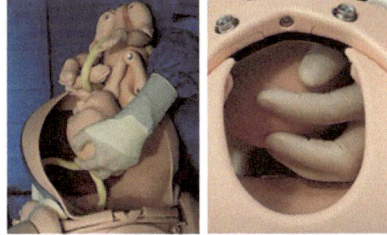

4. Pushing head up

Fig. 11.4 Mechanism of labour during caesarean section

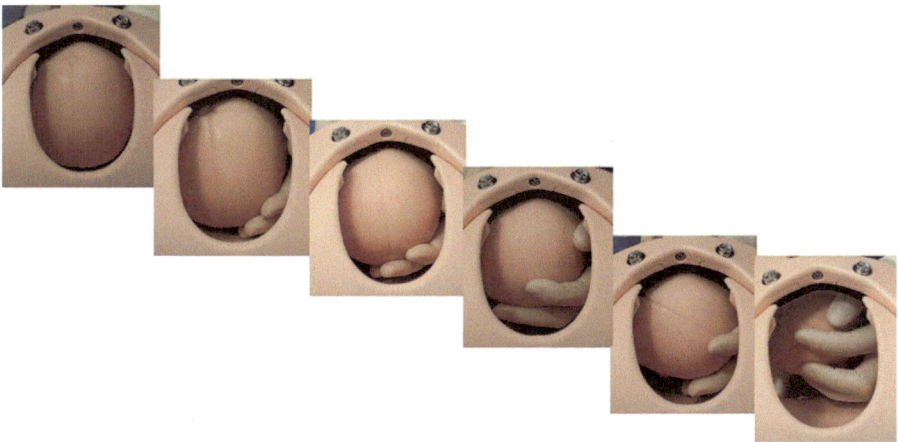

Fig. 11.5 Birth mechanism during caesarean section

11.2.3.3   What to Do Next If You Do Not Manage to Deliver the Baby? [1, 3, 7]

Two methods have been described: the push-and-pull method and the reverse breech extraction. There is no evidence which method should be performed first. In Table 11.1, the advantages and disadvantages of both methods are listed. In short, though the reverse breech extraction may be technically more challenging, it reduces maternal complications, mainly uterotomy tears and blood loss. Neonatal morbidity is higher with the push-and-pull method but neonatal trauma may be similar with both methods. Nevertheless, dramatic complications such as foetal skull fractures and lethal intracranial haemorrhages have been described by using a too firm and localized pressure on the foetal head with the hand and finger pushing up from the vagina. It is important to have a good command of both techniques and have a well-prepared action plan when the baby cannot be delivered with conventional techniques (Table 11.2).

11.2.3.4   Push-and-Pull Method [9]

- First, try a gentle pulling and rotating movement at the foetal shoulders. Sometimes, this will be enough to dislodge the foetal head (Fig. 11.6).
- Then ask an assistant to push the head up from the vagina. Try to push the head up with the palm of your hand as much as possible to avoid localized pressure on the skull by the fingers. At the same time, you should try to flex the foetal head (Fig. 11.7).
- At the same time, the obstetrician should insert a hand under the foetal head to flex, rotate, and push the head up and bring it through the uterotomy.

Table 11.2 Comparison of outcomes between the push-and-pull method and reverse breech extraction [1, 3, 7]

	Method	
Outcome	Push and pull	Reverse breech
Neonatal morbidity	↑	↓
Neonatal trauma	=	=
Intensive neonatal care unit	↑	↓
Uterotomy tears	↑	↓
Maternal blood loss	↑	↓
Endomyometritis (uterine infection)	↑	↓

Fig. 11.6 Gentle pull and rotation at the foetal shoulder

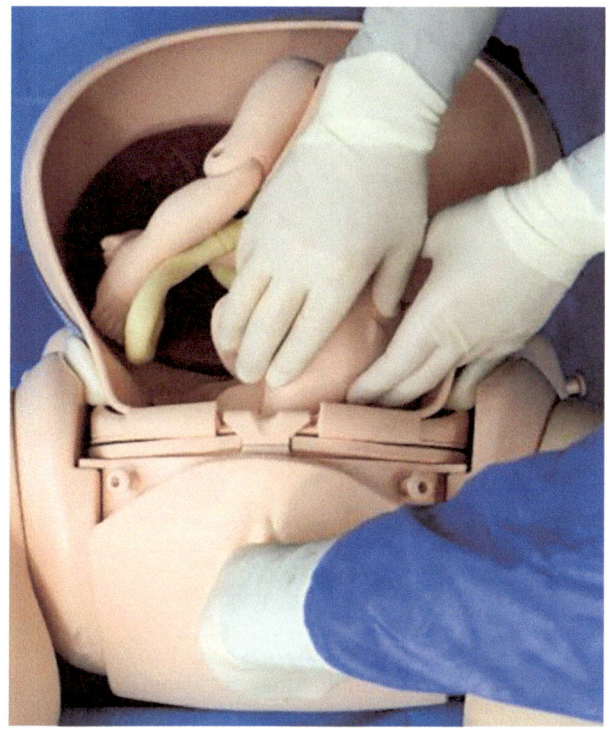

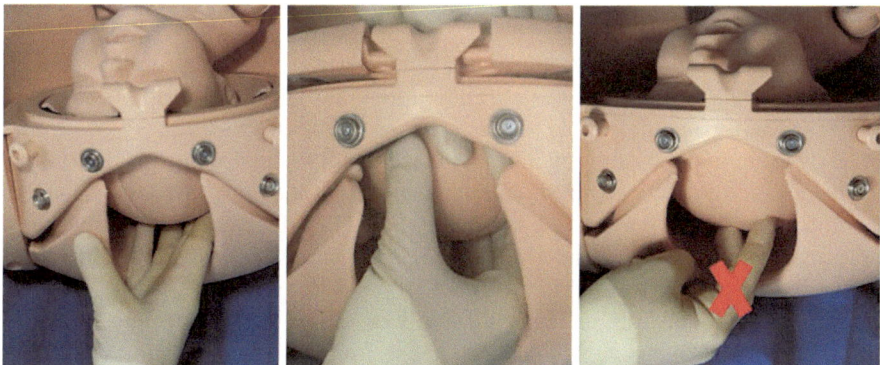

Fig. 11.7 Pushing the foetal head up to the vagina

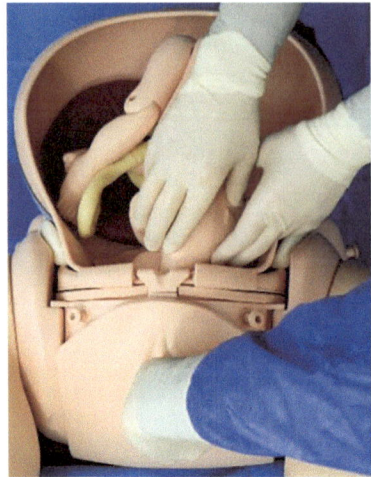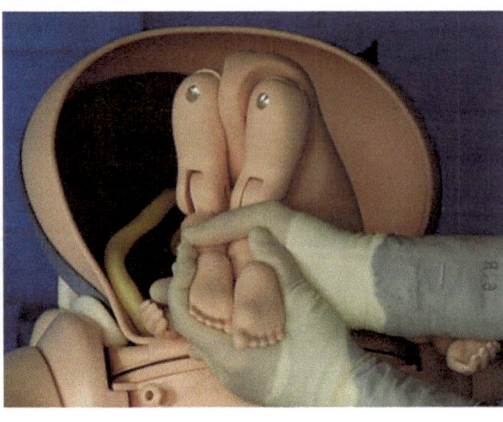

Fig. 11.8 Push-and-pull method and reverse breech extraction

11.2.3.5   Reverse Breech Extraction

In this method, the foetal feet and body are delivered first and the head last (Fig. 11.8). This technique may be technically challenging. Therefore, you should have a clear plan of the steps that have to be achieved to succeed:

- If you managed to easily get both arms through the uterotomy, deliver them. If not, go to the following step. Delivering the arms first was described by Patwardhan et al. and may facilitate delivery of arms and shoulder at the end but is not mandatory.
- Insert your hand inside the uterus and search for one foot or if possible both feet. If you struggle to find the feet, follow the foetal back toward the buttocks and legs. Then, you will be able to grasp at least one foot.
- Extending the uterotomy in a T or J shape is not mandatory. It will increase the risk of uterine rupture in further pregnancies. If you do not have enough space to find a foetal foot, perform the extension (Fig. 11.9). Do not extend the uterotomy further laterally, as this has a high risk of deep parametrium tear, high blood loss, difficult repair, and lesion to the ureter.
- Pull at the foetal foot or feet until the body is delivered. Grasping feet with a towel at this stage may help keep them from slipping through your hands. Meanwhile, your assistant should help by applying pressure on the fundus.
- Help delivering the shoulders and arms if needed.
- To deliver the foetal head, birth mechanics must be respected. This step may be challenging, though. Grasp the baby at the level of the buttocks. Take care not to apply pressure on soft abdominal tissues. Try to gently move the head in an oblique or cross diameter before delivering it. At the end, a Veit–Smellie–Mauriceau manoeuvre to flex the head may be necessary. These steps are illustrated in Fig. 11.10.

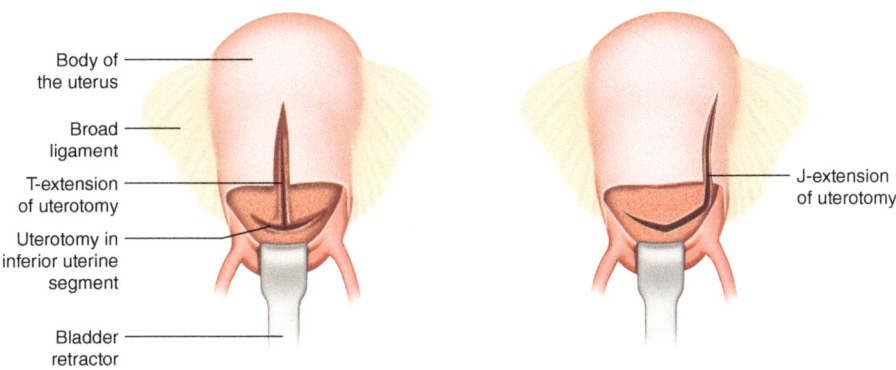

Fig. 11.9 T- or J-shaped extension of uterotomy, if needed to get access to the baby's foot

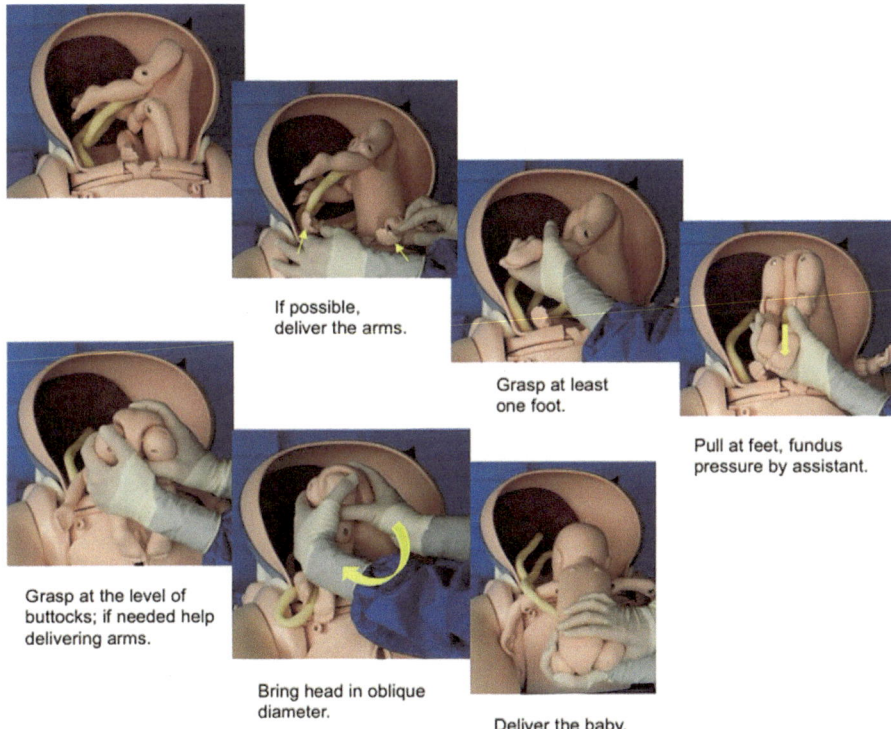

Fig. 11.10 Reverse breech extraction [10]

11.2.4   Actions After Birth of the Baby

- Birth canal examination: search for tears in parametrium and/or cervix/vagina.
- If one cannot get a clear view: Uterus luxation outside abdominal cavity (it will increase the tension on uterine arteries and minimize the bleeding).
- If deep parametrium tear: Take care not to ligate the ureter!
- Examine the baby for injuries.

11.3   Algorithm

Figure 11.11 depicts the algorithm in case of difficult foetal extraction at caesarean section at full dilatation.

Checklist – Difficult fetal extraction at C-Section (CS) with deeply impacted fetal head

Actions preoperative
- Stop oxytocin at CS indication
- Control fetal position (US, Vag. exam.)
- Frog-leg position of mother legs
- **Vaginal examination in OP**: vaginal operative delivery possible?
- Consider device installation (Fetal Pillow/C- Snorkel)
- Team Time Out: PPH/ fetal extraction!

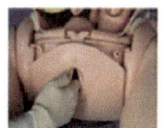

Risk factors
Full dilatation, low fetal presentation (spinae ischiatica)
- Slow birth progress
- Deflexed occipito-posterior cephalic presentation

Actions intraoperative
- Bladder flap
- Uterotomy higher than usual
- Flexion and rotation of the fetal head in the cross diameter
- Access fetal head from the side if no space behind symphysis

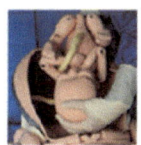 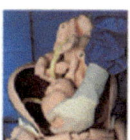

If quick fetal extraction not possible:
- **Call for HELP!** (experienced obstetrician)
- Trendelenburg + Nitroglycerin i.v. (Anesthetist)
- OP-Table low!
- Change hand- or side : left or right hand
- Symmetrical gentle pull upwards on fetal shoulders with concurrent rotation
- If strong uterus contraction wait for 30 s

Reverse breech extraction
- Extract arms first
- Reach for both feet, deliver fetal body, head as last part
- Enlarge uterotomy in T or J shape if space needed

PUSH and PULL Method
- Push fetal head upwards with a vaginal hand, as flat as possible or with silicon vacuum cup.
- Symmetrical gentle pull upwards on fetal shoulders with concurrent rotation
- Enlarge uterotomy in T or J shape if space needed

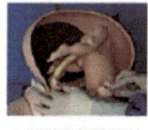 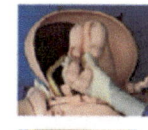

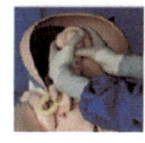 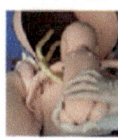

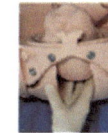 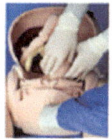

Fig. 11.11 Algorithm: difficult extraction at caesarean section with impacted foetal head (Permission from DeGruyter 2024 [11])

11.4 Conclusion

CSFD may well be a very challenging issue when the foetal head is deeply impacted into the maternal pelvis. Be aware and prepared to quickly perform the extraction manoeuvres to improve outcome of both mother and child.

Models used for the figures:

Birthing Simulator PROMPT Flex—Standard

Enhanced Caesarean Section Module (ECSM)—PROMPT Flex

Laerdal training mannequin BLS

MVB Foetal head obstetrical training model

References

1. Waterfall H, Grivell RM, Dodd JM. Techniques for assisting difficult delivery at caesarean section. Cochrane Database Syst Rev. 2016;2016(1):CD004944.
2. Cornthwaite KR, Bahl R, Lattey K, Draycott T. Management of impacted fetal head at cesarean delivery. Am J Obstet Gynecol. 2024;230(3s):S980–S7.
3. Jeve YB, Navti OB, Konje JC. Comparison of techniques used to deliver a deeply impacted fetal head at full dilation: a systematic review and meta-analysis. BJOG. 2016;123(3):337–45.
4. WHO. Surgical safety checklist.
5. Alexander JM, Leveno KJ, Rouse DJ, Landon MB, Gilbert S, Spong CY, et al. Comparison of maternal and infant outcomes from primary cesarean delivery during the second compared with first stage of labor. Obstet Gynecol. 2007;109(4):917–21.
6. Allen VM, O'Connell CM, Baskett TF. Maternal and perinatal morbidity of caesarean delivery at full cervical dilatation compared with caesarean delivery in the first stage of labour. BJOG. 2005;112(7):986–90.
7. Berhan Y, Berhan A. A meta-analysis of reverse breech extraction to deliver a deeply impacted head during cesarean delivery. Int J Gynaecol Obstet. 2014;124(2):99–105.
8. Loudon JA, Groom KM, Hinkson L, Harrington D, Paterson-Brown S. Changing trends in operative delivery performed at full dilatation over a 10-year period. J Obstet Gynaecol. 2010;30(4):370–5.
9. Landesman R, Graber EA. Abdominovaginal delivery: modification of the cesarean section operation to facilitate delivery of the impacted head. Am J Obstet Gynecol. 1984;148(6):707–10.
10. Patwardhan BD, Motashaw ND. Caesarean section. J Obstet Gynecol India. 1957;8:1–15.
11. Monod C, Buechel J, Gisin S, Abo El Ela A, Vogt DR, Hoesli I. Simulation of an impacted fetal head extraction during cesarean section: description of the creation and evaluation of a new training program. J Perinat Med. 2019;47(8):857–66.
12. Monod C, et al. Reverse breech extraction with the model. 2022.
13. Unterscheider J, McMenamin M, Cullinane F. Rising rates of caesarean deliveries at full cervical dilatation: a concerning trend. Eur J Obstet Gynecol Reprod Biol. 2011;157(2):141–4.
14. Sobhy S, Arroyo-Manzano D, Murugesu N, Karthikeyan G, Kumar V, Kaur I, et al. Maternal and perinatal mortality and complications associated with caesarean section in low-income and middle-income countries: a systematic review and meta-analysis. Lancet. 2019;393(10184):1973–82.
15. Attilakos GDT, Gale A, Siassakos D, Winter C. ROBuST: RCOH Operative birth simulation Training Course Manual. Cambridge University Press. 2013.

Open Access This chapter is licensed under the terms of the Creative Commons Attribution 4.0 International License (http://creativecommons.org/licenses/by/4.0/), which permits use, sharing, adaptation, distribution and reproduction in any medium or format, as long as you give appropriate credit to the original author(s) and the source, provide a link to the Creative Commons license and indicate if changes were made.

The images or other third party material in this chapter are included in the chapter's Creative Commons license, unless indicated otherwise in a credit line to the material. If material is not included in the chapter's Creative Commons license and your intended use is not permitted by statutory regulation or exceeds the permitted use, you will need to obtain permission directly from the copyright holder.

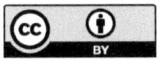

Correction to: Simulation Training for Obstetric Emergencies in Low-Resource Countries

Correction to:
C. Monod et al., *Simulation Training for Obstetric Emergencies in Low-Resource Countries,*
https://doi.org/10.1007/978-3-031-81931-5

This book was inadvertently published with the following errors, which have now been corrected and incorporated into the book.

1. Figure 9.3 should be replaced with an alternative image that was previously produced and discussed.

Incorrect Fig. 9.3 on page 77   Correct Fig. 9.3 to be replaced on page 77

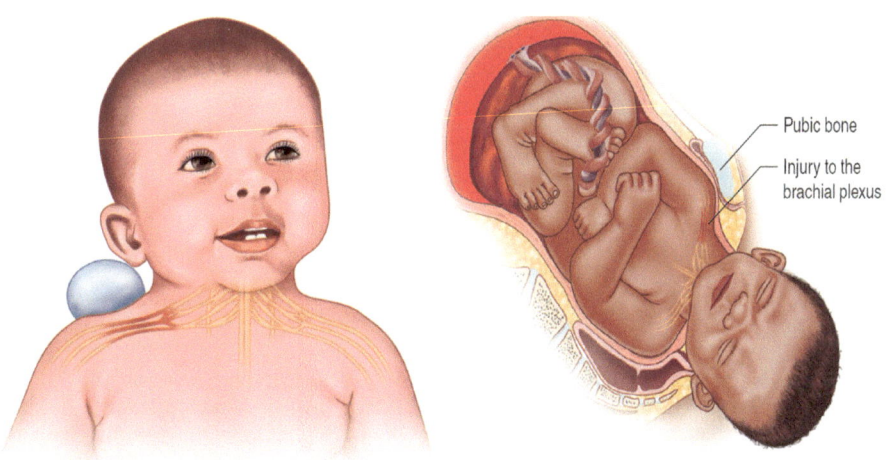

Fig. 9.3 Stretching of brachial plexus nerves in shoulder dystocia

The updated version of this book can be found at
https://doi.org/10.1007/978-3-031-81931-5

© The Author(s) 2025   C1
C. Monod et al., *Simulation Training for Obstetric Emergencies
in Low-Resource Countries*, https://doi.org/10.1007/978-3-031-81931-5_12

2. On page 36, Fig. 4.13 overlapped with the figure legend, and this has been corrected.
3. Video links of Chaps. 5, 10, and 11 were not running and these have been checked.
4. The author names were earlier listed as Cécile Monod, Irene Hoesli, Samira Akra, Martina Gisin, Annkathrin Butenschoen, Stavroula Katsaouni, Lara Sirdey Fiechter, and Katharina Redling, while the correct order of the author names is *Cécile Monod, Irene Hoesli, Martina Gisin, Samira Akra, Annkathrin Butenschoen, Stavroula Katsaouni, Lara Sirdey Fiechter, and Katharina Redling.*

Open Access This chapter is licensed under the terms of the Creative Commons Attribution 4.0 International License (http://creativecommons.org/licenses/by/4.0/), which permits use, sharing, adaptation, distribution and reproduction in any medium or format, as long as you give appropriate credit to the original author(s) and the source, provide a link to the Creative Commons license and indicate if changes were made.

The images or other third party material in this chapter are included in the chapter's Creative Commons license, unless indicated otherwise in a credit line to the material. If material is not included in the chapter's Creative Commons license and your intended use is not permitted by statutory regulation or exceeds the permitted use, you will need to obtain permission directly from the copyright holder.

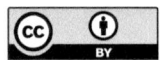

Literature

1. Gordon M, Baker P, Catchpole K, Darbyshire D, Schocken D. Devising a consensus definition and framework for non-technical skills in healthcare to support educational design: a modified Delphi study. Med Teach. 2015;37(6):572–7.
2. Helmreich RL. On error management: lessons from aviation. BMJ. 2000;320(7237):781–5.
3. Haerkens MH, Kox M, Lemson J, Houterman S, van der Hoeven JG, Pickkers P. Crew resource management in the intensive care unit: a prospective 3-year cohort study. Acta Anaesthesiol Scand. 2015;59(10):1319–29.
4. Knight M, Kenyon S, Brocklehurst P, Neilson J, Shakespeare J, Kurinczuk JJ, editors., on behalf of MBRRACEUK. Saving lives, improving mothers' care—Lessons learned to inform future maternity care from the UK and Ireland Confidential Enquiries into Maternal Deaths and Morbidity 2009–2012. Oxford: National Perinatal Epidemiology Unit, University of Oxford; 2014.
5. Simons DJ. Monkeying around with the gorillas in our midst: familiarity with an inattentional-blindness task does not improve the detection of unexpected events. Iperception. 2010;1(1):3–6.
6. Nielsen P, Mann S. Team function in obstetrics to reduce errors and improve outcomes. Obstet Gynecol Clin North Am. 2008;35(1):81–95, ix.
7. Rall MGD. Human performance and patient safety. In: Miller's anesthesia. Philadelphia: Elsevier; 2009. p. 93–150.
8. Haig KM, Sutton S, Whittington J. SBAR: a shared mental model for improving communication between clinicians. Jt Comm J Qual Patient Saf. 2006;32(3):167–75.
9. Team TPE. PROMPT Course Manual, Practical Obstetric Multi-Professional Training. 3rd ed. Cambridge: Cambridge University Press; 2017.
10. Chu J, Johnston TA, Geoghegan J. Maternal collapse in pregnancy and the puerperium: green-top guideline no. 56. BJOG. 2020;127(5):e14–52.
11. Olasveengen TM, Semeraro F, Ristagno G, Castren M, Handley A, Kuzovlev A, et al. European Resuscitation Council guidelines 2021: basic life support. Resuscitation. 2021;161:98–114.
12. Gandhi A, Gandhi A. Cardiopulmonary resuscitation in the pregnant woman. In: Global women's medicine. 2021;13.
13. Burns RD. Managing medical and obstetric emergencies and trauma. In: The MOET course manual. 4rd ed. Cambridge: Cambridge University Press; 2022.
14. WHO. WHO recommendations for the prevention and treatment of postpartum haemorrhage. 2012.
15. Begley CM, Gyte GM, Devane D, McGuire W, Weeks A, Biesty LM. Active versus expectant management for women in the third stage of labour. Cochrane Database Syst Rev. 2019;2(2):CD007412.

© The Editor(s) (if applicable) and The Author(s) 2025   123
C. Monod et al., *Simulation Training for Obstetric Emergencies in Low-Resource Countries*, https://doi.org/10.1007/978-3-031-81931-5

16. https://www.glowm.com/resource-type/resource/textbook/title/a-/title/a-comprehensive-textbook-of-postpartum-hemorrhage-2nd-edition/resource-doc/1275.
17. Queensland Health. Postpartum haemorrhage guideline no. MN18.1V10-R23 2021.
18. Knight M, Bunch K, Felker A, Patel R, Kotnis R, Kenyon S, Kurinczuk JJ. Saving lives, improving mothers' care. MBRRACE-UK. 2023.
19. https://globalhealthmedia.org/videos/uterine-balloon-tamponade/.
20. Dueckelmann AM, Hinkson L, Nonnenmacher A, Siedentopf JP, Schoenborn I, Weizsaecker K, et al. Uterine packing with chitosan-covered gauze compared to balloon tamponade for managing postpartum hemorrhage. Eur J Obstet Gynecol Reprod Biol. 2019;240:151–5.
21. B-Lynch C, Shah H. Conservative surgical management. In: Arulkumaran S, Karoshi M, Keith LG, Lalonde AB, B-Lynch C, editors. A comprehensive textbook of postpartum hemorrhage. 2nd ed. London: Sapiens Publishing; 2012. p. 433–40.
22. B-Lynch C, Keith LG, Campbell WB. Internal Iliac (hypogastric) artery ligation. In: Arulkumaran S, Karoshi M, Keith LG, Lalonde AB, B-Lynch C, editors. A comprehensive textbook of postpartum hemorrhage. 2nd ed. London: Sapiens Publishing; 2012. p. 441–7.
23. Baskett TF. Peripartum hysterectomy. In: Arulkumaran S, Karoshi M, Keith LG, Lalonde AB, B-Lynch C, editors. A comprehensive textbook of postpartum hemorrhage. 2nd ed. London: Sapiens Publishing; 2012. p. 462–5.
24. https://oss-online.ca/knowledge-base/pph-hys/#technique-total-hysterectomy.
25. WHO Guidelines Approved by the Guidelines Review Committee. WHO recommendations on the assessment of postpartum blood loss and use of a treatment bundle for postpartum haemorrhage. Geneva: World Health Organization; 2023.
26. Gallos I, Devall A, Martin J, Middleton L, Beeson L, Galadanci H, et al. Randomized trial of early detection and treatment of postpartum hemorrhage. N Engl J Med. 2023;389(1):11–21.
27. Hoesli I, et al. B-Lynch-uterine suture with a model. 2020.
28. youTube. Uterine inversion_obstetric podcast. Uterine inversion. 2018. https://www.youtube.com/watch?v=bYIPkNfPDUI&t=4s.
29. NICE Guideline. Hypertension in pregnancy: diagnosis and management. 2019.
30. American College of Obstetricians and Gynecologists' Committee on Practice Bulletins—Obstetrics. ACOG practice bulletin no. 203: chronic hypertension in pregnancy. Obstet Gynecol. 2019;133(1):e26–50.
31. World Health Organization. WHO recommendations for prevention and treatment of pre-eclampsia and eclampsia. 2011.
32. Gestational hypertension and preeclampsia: ACOG practice bulletin, number 222. Obstet Gynecol. 2020;135(6):e237–e260.
33. Magee LA, Brown MA, Hall DR, Gupte S, Hennessy A, Karumanchi SA, Kenny LC, McCarthy F, Myers J, Poon LC, Rana S, Saito S, Staff AC, Tsigas E, von Dadelszen P. The 2021 International Society for the Study of Hypertension in Pregnancy classification, diagnosis & management recommendations for international practice. Pregnancy Hypertens. 2022;27:148–69. https://doi.org/10.1016/j.preghy.2021.09.008.
34. Brown MA, Magee LA, Kenny LC, Karumanchi SA, McCarthy FP, Saito S, et al. The hypertensive disorders of pregnancy: ISSHP classification, diagnosis & management recommendations for international practice. Hypertension. 2018;13:291–310.
35. World Health Organization. WHO recommendations: drug treatment for severe hypertension in pregnancy. 2018.
36. WHO. WHO essential medication list 2021. 2021.
37. Magee LA, Nicolaides KH, von Dadelszen P. Preeclampsia. N Engl J Med. 2022;386(19):1817–32.
38. World Health Organization. WHO recommendations, policy of interventionist versus expectant management in severe pre-eclampsia before term. 2018.
39. WHO. WHO statement on maternal sepsis 2017.
40. World Health Organization. WHO recommendations for prevention and treatment of maternal peripartum infections. 2015.
41. Global Maternal and Neonatal Sepsis Initiative. GLOSS the global maternal sepsis study. WHO.

42. Bowyer L, Robinson HL, Barrett H, Crozier TM, Giles M, Idel I, et al. SOMANZ guidelines for the investigation and management sepsis in pregnancy. Aust N Z J Obstet Gynaecol. 2017;57(5):540–51.
43. McNarry AF, Goldhill DR. Simple bedside assessment of level of consciousness: comparison of two simple assessment scales with the Glasgow Coma scale. Anaesthesia. 2004;59(1):34–7.
44. Shields A, de Assis V, Halscott T. Top 10 pearls for the recognition, evaluation, and management of maternal sepsis. Obstet Gynecol. 2021;138(2):289–304.
45. The UK Sepsis Trust. 2020.
46. RCOG. Shoulder dystocia. Green-top guideline no. 42, 2nd ed. 2012.
47. Wikipedia. Brachial plexus. https://en.wikipedia.org/wiki/Brachial_plexus.
48. UCSF Benioff Children's Hospital. Neonatal hypoxic ischemic encephalopathy.
49. Gilstrop M, Hoffman MK. An update on the acute management of shoulder dystocia. Clin Obstet Gynecol. 2016;59(4):813–9.
50. Frontiers Ms. Medical guidelines.
51. Enekwe A, Rothmund R, Uhl B. Abdominal access for shoulder dystocia as a last resort—a case report. Geburtshilfe Frauenheilkd. 2012;72(7):634–8.
52. Operative vaginal birth: ACOG practice bulletin, number 219. Obstet Gynecol. 2020;135(4):e149-e159.
53. Murphy DJ, Strachan BK, Bahl R. Assisted vaginal birth: green-top guideline no. 26. BJOG. 2020;127(9):e70–e112.
54. Attilakos G, Draycott T, Gale A, Siassakos D, Winter C. ROBuST: RCOG operative birth simulation training: course manual. Cambridge: Cambridge University Press; 2013.
55. Vacca Academy. Handbook of vacuum delivery in obstetrics. Brisbane: Vacca Academy; 2009.
56. Laborie. Vacuum assisted delivery proper cup placement. 2022. https://www.laborie.com/education/video-gallery/.
57. Loudon JA, Groom KM, Hinkson L, Harrington D, Paterson-Brown S. Changing trends in operative delivery performed at full dilatation over a 10-year period. J Obstet Gynaecol. 2010;30(4):370–5.
58. Unterscheider J, McMenamin M, Cullinane F. Rising rates of caesarean deliveries at full cervical dilatation: a concerning trend. Eur J Obstet Gynecol Reprod Biol. 2011;157(2):141–4.
59. Sobhy S, Arroyo-Manzano D, Murugesu N, Karthikeyan G, Kumar V, Kaur I, et al. Maternal and perinatal mortality and complications associated with caesarean section in low-income and middle-income countries: a systematic review and meta-analysis. Lancet. 2019;393(10184):1973–82.
60. Waterfall H, Grivell RM, Dodd JM. Techniques for assisting difficult delivery at caesarean section. Cochrane Database Syst Rev. 2016;2016(1):CD004944.
61. Alexander JM, Leveno KJ, Rouse DJ, Landon MB, Gilbert S, Spong CY, et al. Comparison of maternal and infant outcomes from primary cesarean delivery during the second compared with first stage of labor. Obstet Gynecol. 2007;109(4):917–21.
62. Allen VM, O'Connell CM, Baskett TF. Maternal and perinatal morbidity of caesarean delivery at full cervical dilatation compared with caesarean delivery in the first stage of labour. BJOG. 2005;112(7):986–90.
63. Cornthwaite KR, Bahl R, Lattey K, Draycott T. Management of impacted fetal head at cesarean delivery. Am J Obstet Gynecol. 2024;230(3s):S980–7.
64. Jeve YB, Navti OB, Konje JC. Comparison of techniques used to deliver a deeply impacted fetal head at full dilation: a systematic review and meta-analysis. BJOG. 2016;123(3):337–45.
65. WHO. Surgical safety checklist.
66. Berhan Y, Berhan A. A meta-analysis of reverse breech extraction to deliver a deeply impacted head during cesarean delivery. Int J Gynaecol Obstet. 2014;124(2):99–105.
67. Landesman R, Graber EA. Abdominovaginal delivery: modification of the cesarean section operation to facilitate delivery of the impacted head. Am J Obstet Gynecol. 1984;148(6):707–10.
68. Monod C, Buechel J, Gisin S, Abo El Ela A, Vogt DR, Hoesli I. Simulation of an impacted fetal head extraction during cesarean section: description of the creation and evaluation of a new training program. J Perinat Med. 2019;47(8):857–66.
69. Monod C, et al. Reverse breech extraction with the model. 2022.